allergy free

COOKBOOK FOR THE FAMILY

allergy free

COOKBOOK FOR THE FAMILY

Brianna Monson

BONNEVILLE BOOKS

SPRINGVILLE, UTAH

ISBN 13: 978-1-59955-458-7

Published by Bonneville Books an imprint of Cedar Fort, Inc., 2373 W. 700 S., Springville, UT 84663
Distributed by Cedar Fort, Inc., www.cedarfort.com

LIBRARY OF CONGRESS CATALOGING-IN-PUBLICATION DATA

Monson, Brianna.
  Allergy free for the family / Brianna Monson.
    p. cm.
  Includes index.
  ISBN 978-1-59955-458-7
  1. Cookery--United States. 2. Food allergy--Diet therapy--Recipes. I.
Title.

  RM219.M575 2010
  641.5'631--dc22

2010026018

Cover design and typesetting by Danie Romrell
Cover design © 2010 by Lyle Mortimer
Edited by Melissa J. Caldwell

Printed in China

10 9 8 7 6 5 4 3 2 1

Printed on acid-free paper

Dedication

To Michael and Arianna—

May these recipes bless your lives for many
years to come.

Contents

Drinks

Side Dishes

Snacks

Soups

Acknowledgments

To my husband, thank you for your love and support. To my children, thank you for tasting my creations and helping in the kitchen. To Mom and Dad, thank you for making your home allergy friendly. To Mom, thank you for helping cook for all the photographs in the cookbook. To Grandma, thank you for writing a poem that illustrates your understanding. To Jenne, thank you for your photography expertise and the beautiful pictures.

Introduction

I know that if you are reading this book, you have a desire to find some allergy-free recipes for yourself or a loved one. I hope these recipes will help all those that have opened this book! As a mother of a child with life-threatening food allergies, I have experienced firsthand how food allergies can exclude the allergy sufferer from participating in family or social gatherings involving food. Determined to allow my son to feel included, I experimented to create safe recipes our whole family can enjoy. I'm grateful for the opportunity to create these recipes for my family. I know that you'll benefit from this book and value it in your everyday life.

My grandmother wrote the following poem, and it means a lot to me. I love how it really conveys the message of what life is truly like for an allergy sufferer or the family. I know you will enjoy it too.

Allergy Challenge

My dreams of marriage and family were beginning to come true.
With happiness and love and skies always blue.
When a wee babe was placed in our loving arms
He captured our hearts with his sweet baby charms.
But it soon became apparent that he had special needs
Life-threatening allergies—frightening indeed!
In my eyes the task loomed great.
Making the foods he could tolerate.
No wheat, no milk, no deadly eggs—what was left?
Research and study left me bereft.
I determined to do all within my power
So we could each enjoy the dinner hour.
Through trial and error, testing and waste
I created safe foods that please our taste.
From my Family Friendly Recipes I'm sure you will make
Crackers and meatloaf, ice cream and cake!

—written by Phyllis Rose

Just a Little Advice

As you begin this journey of allergen-free/gluten-free cooking, you will feel a bit overwhelmed. Be sure to take your time and read every recipe carefully before you begin.

Decide which ingredients you need to purchase. Most grocery stores are beginning to carry more and more specialty foods. If you cannot find what you need at your grocer, check a health food store. If you still need help, there are many online resources (see resources section p. 102).

Don't worry too much if your finished product doesn't always look perfect or look the way you may be used to. The food will taste great regardless. Remember, it may take a little practice if you are just starting out.

Be sure to place cookie dough in your refrigerator for one hour before baking. This will really help in the finished product, and the cookie will stay together and look great.

Prepare Your Pantry

When my son was first diagnosed with food allergies, I realized how expensive buying allergen free would be. I was determined to create recipes within a budget, using products that I could find. It may be a bit more time consuming to bake from the ground up, but, believe me, it is well worth it for many reasons: tastes great, costs less, and is healthier.

If you keep ingredients in your pantry, you'll be ready to make a great meal or bake a tasty treat at any moment. Please make sure you read every label, check with your allergist, and call the manufacturer to ensure the safety of your foods. Many products change without notice, and ingredients do too, so ALWAYS read labels before you begin. On the following page is a list of some of the less familiar ingredients in this book, a short description, and where they can be purchased.

Ingredient Hints

Chicken Broth—I use Pacific brand (www.pacificfoods.com).

Cocoa—Please be sure to purchase an all-natural cocoa without dairy.

Coconut Flakes—I use shredded coconut, but please check with your doctor if you have a tree nut allergy to be safe.

Corn and Rice Cereals—There are a lot of cereals to choose from, so just be sure to check labels and manufacturing information. We use Rice Krispies, Kix, Corn Flakes, Corn Chex, and Rice Chex.

Dairy-free Chocolate Chips—I use Enjoy Life brand (www.enjoylifefood.com).

Dairy-free Cream Cheese—I use Tofutti brand (www.tofutti.com)

Dairy-free Creamer—I use Silk brand (www.silksoymilk.com).

Dairy-free Margarine—A wonderful alternative to dairy margarine or traditional butter. There are many brands on the market. I use Nucoa, Earth Balance, and Vegan Smart Balance brands (www.earthbalancenatural.com, www.smartbalance.com).

Dairy-free Shortening—I use Crisco at times and also Spectrum, which is soy free too. So, depending on your needs you have a few choices.

Dairy-free Whipped Topping—I use Soy Whip. This is great to add on top of a pie, hot cocoa, or Italian soda (www.spectrumorganics.com).

Egg Replacer—When you can't have an egg and you need a substitute, this is great. I use the Ener-G brand (www.ener-g.com).

Guar Gum—I use this ingredient in one recipe (Corn Dog Bites). I attempted over and over to create a corn dog, and they would just fall apart. So, I tried adding guar gum after a little research, and it held together (www.authenticfoods.com, www.bobsredmill.com).

Hot Dogs—I use original Oscar Mayer brand.

Marshmallows—Be sure to find gluten-free and egg-free. I use Kraft brand.

Oat Flour—If you have a gluten-free diet, you will want to be sure to find the certified gluten-free oats that are now available. To make oat flour, pour oats into a blender or food processor and grate until flour is fine. If you do not need a gluten-free diet, you can purchase prepackaged oat flour.

Oil—I use corn oil or canola oil a lot in baking. But be sure you check the ingredients. I also use olive oil at times when I fry or sauté dishes.

Potato Flour—This is not the same as potato starch. Be sure to use potato flour.

Rice Flour—This is very easy to find. It's just ground up rice, so if you have a grinder you may choose to make your own.

Soy Milk—I use vanilla soy milk in my recipes because I like the flavor. But you can use plain soy milk, rice milk, or cow's milk in equal measure.

Soy Milk Powder—I find this at my local health food store but if your local health food store doesn't carry it, you can purchase it through an online retailer.

Soy Nut Butter—This is the peanut-free version of peanut butter that my children love.

Soy Sauce—Be sure to find a gluten-free brand. I use San-J (www.san-j.com).

Tapioca Starch or Tapioca Flour—These two flours are the same, so whichever you find will work (www.ener-g.com).

Vanilla—Be sure to find a brand that is gluten free.

Xanthan Gum—This great ingredient is very helpful in non-gluten recipes to help the products rise. I use Ener-G brand but be sure to check the ingredients (www.ener-g.com).

Substitutions

Eggs—I use Ener-G Egg Replacer in my recipes. If you can tolerate eggs, you may substitute 1 egg for every 1½ teaspoon of egg replacer and 2 tablespoons warm water.

Milk—I use soy milk. If your diet does not allow soy you may substitute rice or cow's milk in equal measure. You may need to adjust the measurements slightly based on thickness and taste preference. I find that rice milk makes things thinner and soy milk makes things taste sweeter.

Margarine and Shortening—Be sure to find a suitable alternative to traditional margarine and shortening. There are many dairy-free margarines on the market. There is also shortening that is soy and dairy free. More local grocery stores are starting to carry these items, but if your grocery store doesn't carry them, you can find them at a health food store.

Oil—Be sure to check the ingredients in the oil you usually use. Some oils are made with soybean oil, so find an oil that you can safely consume, and have it available for your recipes.

Flour—I use a variety of flours in the recipes. If you do not have a wheat allergy, you may substitute a flour of your choice in equal measure.

Symbol Key

After each recipe, the following symbols indicate the different allergens:

E   D   S   T   N   SH   F   W   G

E = egg   SH = shellfish

D = dairy   F = fish

S = soy   W = wheat

T = tree nut   G = gluten

N = nut

Dark-colored letters indicate what the recipe is free of while light-colored letters indicate what the recipe still contains. I have also included variations of the recipe before the symbols if there is a remaining allergen.

Note: The recipes in this book are those that the author feeds her family. Every attempt has been made to ensure the information contained herein is as accurate as possible. She is not a doctor, an allergist, or a dietician. The author assumes no responsibility for damages, injury, or other consequence resulting from use of information contained in this book. If you think you suffer from food allergies, please consult your health care provider.

Breads

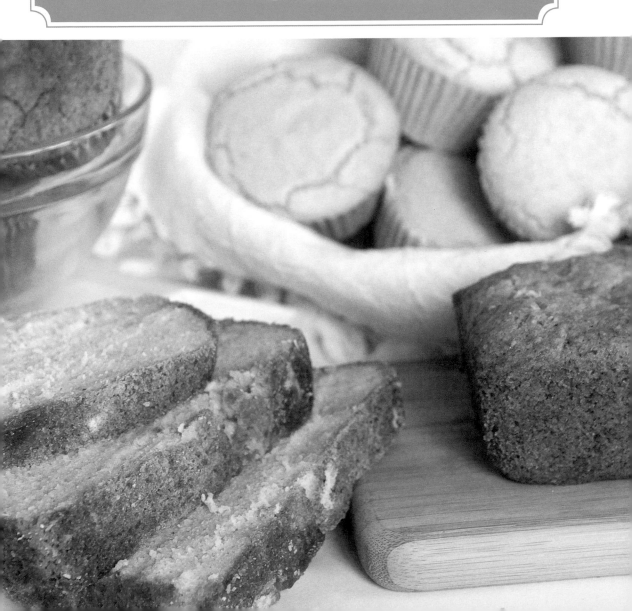

breads

Banana Bread

I always have extra bananas, so I had to come up with a banana bread recipe. Every time I make banana bread or banana muffins, they're gone that day.

1¼ cups bananas (2 bananas), mashed
½ tsp. vanilla (gluten free)
¾ cup sugar
¼ cup oil
1 Tbsp. dairy-free margarine
1 tsp. cream of tartar
1 tsp. baking soda
1 cup rice flour
¼ cup oat flour

MIX bananas, vanilla, and sugar. Add oil and margarine, and mix. Add cream of tartar, baking soda, rice flour, and oat flour. Mix until well blended. Pour into a greased 8 x 4 x 2 loaf pan, and bake at 350 degrees for 30–35 minutes. To make muffins, pour into muffin cups ¾ full and bake at 350 degrees for 20–25 minutes. Makes 12–15 muffins.

Tip: To make oat flour, grate quick oats in blender until flour is fine.
To make this recipe soy free: Substitute dairy-free margarine with an equal amount of soy-free margarine.
To make this recipe gluten free: Substitute oat flour with an equal amount of gluten-free oat flour.

E   D   S   T   N   SH   F   W   G

Cinnamon Muffins

I created these so I could have another type of muffin for my kids to enjoy. They're quick and easy to make and great to put in a school lunch.

½ cup dairy-free margarine
1 Tbsp. oil
½ tsp. cinnamon
½ tsp. salt
1 cup sugar
1 cup applesauce
1 cup rice flour
½ cup oat flour
½ cup tapioca starch
½ tsp. baking soda
½ tsp. cream of tartar

COMBINE all ingredients and mix for 3 minutes. Pour into muffin cups ¾ full and bake at 350 degrees for 20–22 minutes. Makes 18 muffins.

To make this recipe soy free: Substitute dairy-free margarine with an equal amount of soy-free margarine.
To make this recipe gluten free: Substitute oat flour with an equal amount of gluten-free oat flour.

E   D   S   T   N   SH   F   W   G

breads

Gluten-Free Banana Muffins

This is a great gluten-free variation of the banana bread recipe.

1¼ cups bananas, mashed (2 bananas)
½ tsp. vanilla (gluten free)
¾ cup sugar
¼ cup oil
1 tsp. cream of tartar
1 tsp. baking soda
1 cup rice flour
¼ cup tapioca starch

MIX bananas, vanilla, sugar, and oil. Add cream of tartar, baking soda, rice flour, and tapioca starch, and mix until well blended. Pour into muffin cups ¾ full and bake at 350 degrees for 18–20 minutes. Makes 12–15 muffins. To make banana bread, pour into greased 8 x 4 x 2 loaf pan and bake at 350 degrees for 30–35 minutes.

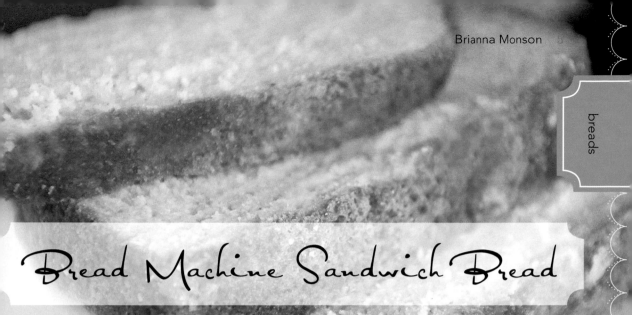

Bread Machine Sandwich Bread

This was my second recipe I created. I wanted to make sandwiches, but my son would spit out all the other bread recipes I tried. This one is super yummy, and my son always wants me to make it.

1½ cups rice flour

1 cup oat flour

1 cup tapioca starch

1 Tbsp. yeast

¼ cup sugar

2 tsp. xanthan gum

1 tsp. salt

1 cup soy milk

¾ cup water

¼ cup dairy-free margarine

2 tsp. egg replacer plus 2 Tbsp. warm water (mix in a bowl first before adding to machine)

2 Tbsp. vinegar

PUT ingredients in your bread machine in the order listed. Program machine to cook a 2-pound, white, medium darkness loaf.

Tip: Keep bread in airtight container. Best if used in a couple days.

To make this recipe soy free: Substitute dairy-free margarine with an equal amount of soy-free margarine. Also substitute soy milk with an equal amount of rice or cow's milk.

To make this recipe gluten free: Substitute oat flour with an equal amount of gluten-free oat flour.

E   D   S   T   N   SH   F   W   G

Dinner Rolls

These are so yummy and won't last long at dinner!

1½ cups rice flour

1 Tbsp. yeast

2 tsp. xanthan gum

1¼ cups soy milk

¼ cup sugar

¼ cup dairy-free margarine

3 tsp. egg replacer plus 4 Tbsp. warm water

2 Tbsp. vinegar

2 cups tapioca starch

1 tsp. salt

COMBINE rice flour, yeast, and xanthan gum in a mixer. Add soy milk, sugar, and margarine, and mix for 30 seconds. In a small bowl, mix egg replacer and warm water thoroughly, and combine with other ingredients. Add vinegar and mix for 1 minute. Add tapioca starch and salt, and knead for 10 minutes. Place dough in a bowl and cover with plastic wrap. Let rise for 2 hours. Grease a cookie sheet and drop dough by spoonfuls onto cookie sheet. Let rise for 2 hours, and bake at 350 degrees for 10–12 minutes. Makes 30 golf ball–sized rolls.

BREAD LOAF VARIATION: Divide dough into 2 equal parts and place in separate loaf pans. Bake at 350 degrees for 25–30 minutes.

CINNAMON TWIST VARIATION: Divide dough into 12 portions. Take each portion and make 2 ropes. Pinch one end of each rope to the other and twist dough ropes together. Melt 4 tablespoons dairy-free margarine and pour on top of twists. Sprinkle cinnamon sugar on top and bake at 350 degrees for 10–12 minutes.

BREADSTICK VARIATION: Divide dough into 12 portions. Take each portion and form into a mini breadstick (3 inches long), and place on cookie sheet. Melt 4 tablespoons dairy-free margarine and pour onto breadsticks. Sprinkle with garlic salt, if desired. Bake at 350 degrees for 10–12 minutes.

HAMBURGER OR HOT DOG BUN VARIATION: Divide dough into 7 portions. Take each portion and form into bun shape. Bake at 350 degrees for 10–15 minutes.

To make this recipe soy free: Substitute dairy-free margarine with an equal amount of soy-free margarine or shortening. Also substitute soy milk with an equal amount of rice or cow's milk.

E   D   S   T   N   SH   F   W   G

Pizza Dough

Pizza is a great Saturday meal. My whole family pitches in to help with all the toppings.

1½ cups warm water
2 Tbsp. yeast
3½ Tbsp. sugar
2 cups rice flour
1 cup oat flour
½ cup tapioca starch
½ cup quick oats
2 tsp. salt
2 tsp. xanthan gum
3 tsp. egg replacer plus 4 Tbsp. warm water
2 Tbsp. oil
1 tsp. vinegar

IN a bowl combine water, yeast, and sugar. Let sit for 5 minutes. In a mixer, combine flours, tapioca starch, oats, salt, and xanthan gum. In separate bowl, mix egg replacer and warm water thoroughly. Stir oil and vinegar into egg replacer. Combine all ingredients and mix for 2 minutes. Place dough in a bowl and cover with plastic wrap. Let rise for 2 hours. Roll into desired pizza shape and place on pizza pan or cookie sheet. Spread oil on top, and sprinkle with garlic salt, and bake at 350 degrees for 20 minutes. Add favorite toppings and bake an additional 20–25 minutes. Makes one medium-sized pizza.

VARIATION: Make pizza breadsticks by dividing dough into 12 portions. Roll into breadstick shape and place on cookie sheet. Spread oil on top and sprinkle with garlic salt. Bake at 350 degrees for 12–15 minutes.

To make this recipe gluten free: Substitute oat flour with an equal amount of gluten-free oat flour. Also, substitute quick oats with an equal amount of gluten-free oats.

E   D   S   T   N   SH   F   W   G

Biscuits

Quick and easy, these biscuits go great with any meal and work well for little sandwiches too.

½ cup rice flour
¼ cup tapioca starch
1 tsp. potato flour
¼ cup cornstarch
1 tsp. xanthan gum
½ tsp. cream of tartar
¼ tsp. baking soda
½ tsp. salt
2 Tbsp. oil
½ cup water

MIX all ingredients in a bowl, adding water last. The dough is ready when you can form it into a ball. Roll out dough onto a rice-floured surface. Cut into biscuit shapes. Bake at 375 degrees for 10 minutes. Makes 1 dozen.

Tip: These are great with dairy-free margarine and jam!

E   D   S   T   N   SH   F   W   G

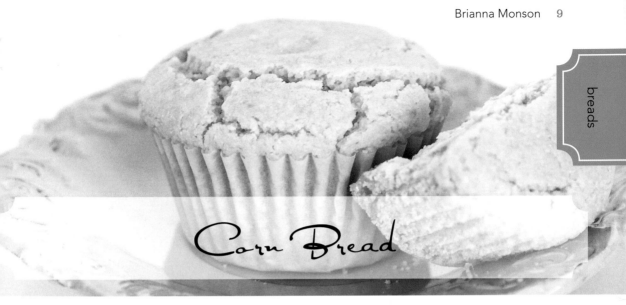

Corn Bread

My family loves this with dairy-free margarine and honey. It's great as a side dish or a treat.

½ cup rice flour
¼ cup tapioca starch
¼ cup cornstarch
1 tsp. potato flour
1 cup cornmeal
1½ tsp. cream of tartar
¾ tsp. baking soda
½ tsp. salt
¼ cup sugar
1 cup soy milk
¼ cup oil

COMBINE all dry ingredients and mix well. Add wet ingredients and stir until well blended. Pour mixture into a greased 8 x 8 pan. Bake at 375 degrees for 18–20 minutes.

Tip: To make into muffins, pour batter into muffin cups ¾ full and bake at 350 degrees for 20–25 minutes. To make this recipe soy free: Substitute soy milk with an equal amount of rice or cow's milk.

E   D   S   T   N   SH   F   W   G

Breakfasts

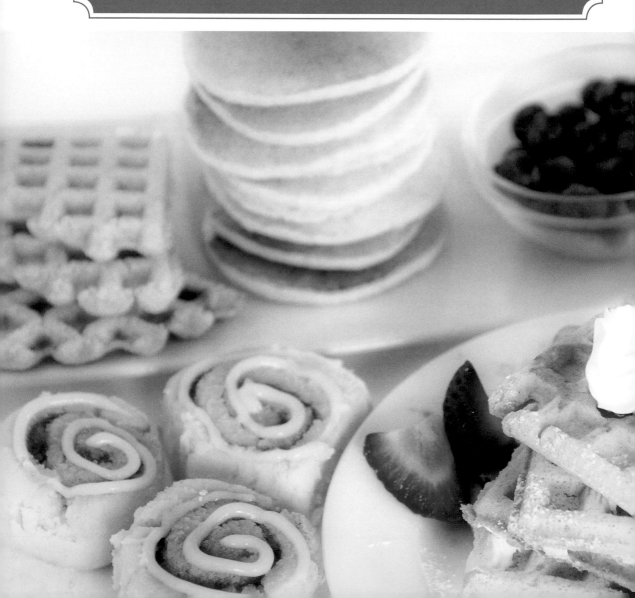

Cinnamon Rolls

I had to create a cinnamon roll that everyone would enjoy. These are so great and worth the effort.

½ Tbsp. yeast

¼ cup warm water

¼ cup shortening

½ cup hot soy milk

½ tsp. salt

¼ cup sugar

¼ cup mashed potatoes, prepared
  (recipe on p. 80)

1½ tsp. Ener-G egg replacer plus 2 Tbsp. water

1½ cups rice flour

1 cup tapioca starch

2 Tbsp. dairy-free margarine

¼ cup sugar

½ tsp. cinnamon

DISSOLVE yeast in warm water and set aside. Stir shortening into hot soy milk until melted and add to mixer. Mix in salt, sugar, and mashed potatoes. When cool, add yeast and stir 1 minute. In a bowl, mix egg replacer and warm water thoroughly, and combine with other ingredients. Add rice flour and tapioca starch. Knead very well (about 10 minutes). Form dough into ball and place in a bowl and cover. Let rise until doubled. Roll dough in a rectangular shape ¼-inch thick on floured surface. Brush with 2 tablespoons melted dairy-free margarine. Mix ¼ cup sugar and ½ tsp. cinnamon and sprinkle over buttered dough. Roll dough up, beginning at wide side. Cut in 1-inch slices and place in a greased pie pan. Let rise for 1 hour and bake at 400 degrees for 10–15 minutes. Makes 16 rolls.

Tip: Tastes great with cream cheese frosting (see p. 24).
To make this recipe soy free: Substitute the dairy-free margarine and shortening with an equal amount of soy-free margarine and shortening. Also substitute soy milk with an equal amount of rice or cow's milk.

E   D   S   T   N   SH   F   W   G

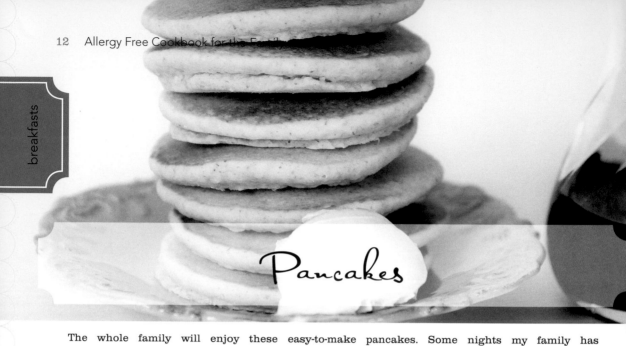

Pancakes

The whole family will enjoy these easy-to-make pancakes. Some nights my family has a breakfast dinner!

¾ cup oat flour
¾ cup rice flour
3 Tbsp. sugar
½ tsp. cream of tartar
¼ tsp. baking soda
½ tsp. salt
1 tsp. lemon juice
1 cup soy milk
1 Tbsp. oil

COMBINE all ingredients in a bowl and stir well. Preheat skillet over medium heat. When hot, pour batter onto frying pan by spoonfuls and cook each side for 2–3 minutes. Serve with favorite toppings. Makes 8–10 medium pancakes.

To make this recipe gluten free: Substitute oat flour with an equal amount of gluten-free oat flour.
To make this recipe soy free: Substitute soy milk with an equal amount of rice or cow's milk.

E   D   S   T   N   SH   F   W   G

Oatmeal Pancakes

These are easy enough for the kids to make.

1½ cups quick oats
1 tsp. potato flour
¼ cup sugar
2 Tbsp. oil
1 tsp. vanilla (gluten free)
1 cup boiling water

COMBINE oats, potato flour, sugar, oil, and vanilla in a bowl. Boil water and add to oat mixture. Stir. Heat skillet over medium heat. When hot, drop oat mixture onto pan by spoonfuls, and cook each side for 3 minutes. Serve with favorite toppings. Makes 8–10 medium pancakes.

To make this recipe gluten free: Substitute quick oats with an equal amount of gluten-free oats.

E   D   S   T   N   SH   F   W   G

Gluten-Free Pancakes

If you can't tolerate oats, here is the pancake for you.

1¼ cups rice flour
3 Tbsp. sugar
½ tsp. cream of tartar
¼ tsp. baking soda
½ tsp. salt
1 tsp. lemon juice
1 cup soy milk
1 Tbsp. oil
¼ tsp. vanilla (gluten free)

COMBINE all ingredients in a bowl and stir well. Heat skillet over medium heat. When hot, drop mixture onto pan by spoonfuls, and cook each side 2–3 minutes. Serve with favorite toppings. Makes 8–10 medium pancakes.

To make this recipe soy free: Substitute soy milk with an equal amount of rice or cow's milk.

E   D   S   T   N   SH   F   W   G

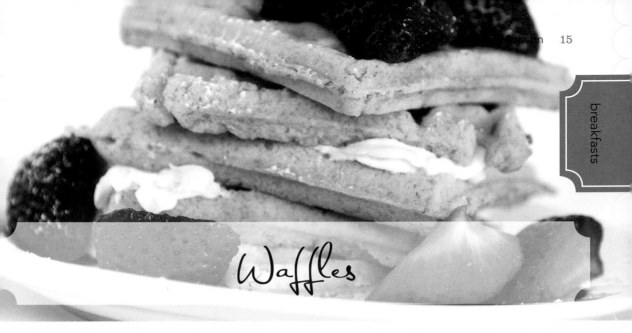

Waffles

I love waffles, and these are fantastic! We love to top our waffles with syrup and strawberries, raspberries, or any other berries that we have on hand.

¾ cup oat flour
¾ cup rice flour
3 Tbsp. sugar
½ tsp. cream of tartar
¼ tsp. baking soda
½ tsp. salt
1 tsp. lemon juice
1⅓ cups soy milk
2 Tbsp. oil

COMBINE all ingredients in a bowl and stir well. Spray waffle iron with dairy-free and gluten-free cooking oil. Pour ⅔ cup of batter onto heated waffle iron and bake. Makes 4 waffles.

To make this recipe gluten free: Substitute oat flour with an equal amount of gluten-free oat flour. To make this recipe soy free: Substitute soy milk with an equal amount of rice or cow's milk. Also, substitute the cooking oil with a soy-free cooking oil.

E   D   S   T   N   SH   F   W   G

Pancake Syrup

I wanted to create a syrup that would go great with the pancakes and waffles on the previous pages. For variety, you can even substitute the vanilla for another flavor.

½ cup corn syrup
½ tsp. vanilla (gluten free)
¼ cup sugar
2 Tbsp. water

MIX all ingredients in pan and heat until boiling. Pour over pancakes.

E   D   S   T   N   SH   F   W   G

Breakfast Burritos

Make extra to freeze. Great for a quick breakfast on the run.

1 (16-oz.) package bacon (dairy and gluten free)
4 cups (6 potatoes) washed, peeled, and diced
1 small green pepper, cut into small pieces
1 cup onion, chopped
1 tsp. salt
¼ tsp. pepper
12 corn or brown rice tortillas

COOK bacon in frying pan on medium heat until done. Crumble bacon into a bowl and set aside. Add potatoes to frying pan with bacon grease. Add green pepper, onion, salt, and pepper. Cook until tender. Place all ingredients into bowl with bacon and stir. Spoon ¼ cup of mixture onto tortillas and fold like a burrito.

E   D   S   T   N   SH   F   W   G

Country Hash Browns

My kids love it when dad is home to make these for breakfast.

½ cup onion, chopped
2 cloves garlic, minced
2 Tbsp. oil
5 potatoes, grated
salt and pepper, to taste

SAUTÉ onion and garlic in a frying pan with oil. Wash and grate potatoes, and add to frying pan. Cook until browned. Add salt and pepper to taste.

E   D   S   T   N   SH   F   W   G

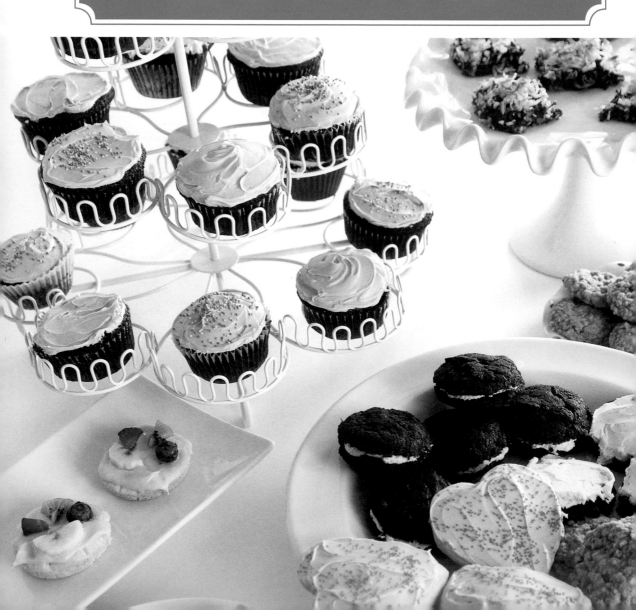

Desserts

Chocolate Chip Cookies

What a great little cookie. We use this cookie to make ice cream sandwiches.

½ cup dairy-free margarine
¼ cup shortening
1 cup brown sugar
½ cup sugar
1 tsp. vanilla (gluten free)
1½ tsp. egg replacer plus 2 Tbsp. warm water
1 cup rice flour
½ cup tapioca starch
½ cup cornstarch
½ Tbsp. potato flour
½ tsp. baking soda
1 tsp. salt
¾ cup dairy-free chocolate chips

MIX margarine, shortening, sugars, and vanilla until smooth. In a small bowl, mix egg replacer and warm water thoroughly. Add to mixture. Add remaining ingredients and mix for 2 minutes. Refrigerate dough for 1 hour. Drop by teaspoonfuls onto ungreased cookie sheet. Bake at 350 degrees for 10–12 minutes. Let cool 2–3 minutes before removing from cookie sheet. Makes 3 dozen.

To make this recipe soy free: Substitute the dairy-free margarine and shortening with an equal amount of soy-free margarine and shortening.

E   D   S   T   N   SH   F   W   G

Chocolate Chip Oatmeal Cookies

This was my first recipe I made allergy free. I grew up making chocolate chip oatmeal cookies with my dad on Sundays. I knew I couldn't have my kids grow up without them, so I had to start here. Everyone that tastes them loves them.

1 cup dairy-free margarine
½ cup shortening
1 cup sugar
2 cups brown sugar
½ cup water
2 tsp. vanilla (gluten free)
3 tsp. egg replacer plus 4 Tbsp. warm water
½ cup tapioca starch

½ cup cornstarch
1 cup rice flour
1½ Tbsp. potato flour
2 tsp. salt
1 tsp. baking soda
6 cups quick oats
1 cup dairy-free chocolate chips

MIX margarine, shortening, sugars, water, and vanilla until smooth. In a small bowl, mix egg replacer and warm water thoroughly. Add to mixture. Add tapioca starch, cornstarch, flours, salt, and baking soda and mix well. Add oats and chocolate chips and mix. Refrigerate dough for 1 hour. Bake at 350 degrees for 10 minutes. Let cool 2–3 minutes before removing from cookie sheet. Makes 6 dozen cookies.

Tip: This dough freezes well. Freeze dough in balls and bake as needed.
To make this recipe soy free: Substitute dairy-free margarine and shortening with an equal amount of soy-free margarine and shortening.
To make this recipe gluten free: Substitute quick oats with an equal amount of gluten-free oats.

E   D   S   T   N   SH   F   W   G

Chocolate Frosted Cookies

This cookie was truly inspired by the traditional Oreo cookie. I wanted a cookie that had yummy frosting inside a chocolaty cookie!

Cookie:

¾ cup dairy-free margarine

1¼ cups sugar

¼ cup dairy-free chocolate chips

3 tsp. egg replacer plus 4 Tbsp. warm water

½ cup cocoa (dairy free)

1 cup rice flour

½ cup tapioca starch

½ tsp. salt

⅛ tsp. cream of tartar

1 tsp. baking soda

Frosting:

¼ cup dairy-free margarine

¼ cup shortening

1⅔ cups powdered sugar

2 tsp. vanilla (gluten free)

TO make the cookie, mix margarine and sugar in a mixer. Melt chocolate chips and add to butter mixture. In a small bowl, mix egg replacer and warm water thoroughly. Add all ingredients together and mix for 3 minutes. Refrigerate dough for 1 hour. Bake at 350 degrees for 10 minutes. Leave on cookie sheet for 2 minutes to cool. To make frosting, mix all ingredients for 3 minutes until smooth. Frost tops of cookies when cookies are cool. Makes 3 dozen cookies.

To make this recipe soy free: Substitute dairy-free margarine and shortening with an equal amount of soy-free margarine and shortening.

E   D   S   T   N   SH   F   W   G

desserts

Sugar Cookies

As a child I would make cut out cookies with my great-grandmother. I loved going to her house and making these cookies—it was such a fun tradition. This is my favorite recipe so far because it rolls out so wonderfully for any holiday cookie. Nobody can tell they are allergen free!

1 cup sugar

½ cup shortening

½ cup dairy-free margarine

3 tsp. egg replacer plus 4 Tbsp. warm water

½ Tbsp. vanilla (gluten free)

1 cup rice flour

¾ cup cornstarch

¾ cup tapioca starch

2 tsp. potato flour

½ tsp. cream of tartar

¼ tsp. baking soda

1 tsp. salt

COMBINE sugar, shortening, and margarine in mixer. In a small bowl, mix egg replacer and warm water thoroughly. Add egg replacer mixture and vanilla to sugar mixture, and mix 1 minute. Add remaining ingredients, and mix until well blended. Refrigerate dough for 1 hour. Roll dough to desired thickness onto hard surface dusted with rice flour. Cut into shapes and bake at 350 degrees for 10 minutes. Let sit on cookie sheet for 2 minutes, and cool completely before frosting (see recipe p. 24). Makes approximately 3 dozen cookies.

To make this recipe soy free: Substitute dairy-free margarine and shortening with an equal amount of soy-free margarine and shortening.

E   D   S   T   N   SH   F   W   G

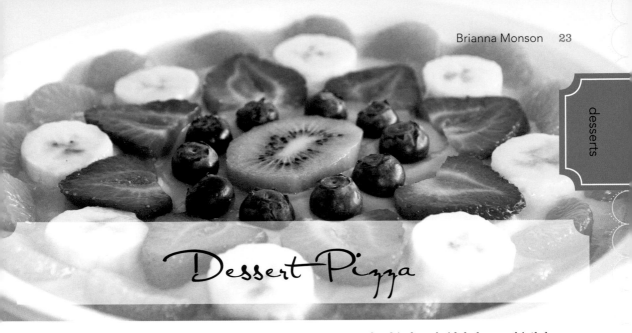

Dessert Pizza

Dessert pizzas are so fun to make and delicious too! You can make this for a bridal shower, birthday party, or just because. Before I came up with a cake recipe, I made a dessert pizza in place of a birthday cake.

1 cup sugar

½ cup shortening

½ cup dairy-free margarine

3 tsp. egg replacer plus 4 Tbsp. warm water

½ Tbsp. vanilla (gluten free)

1 cup rice flour

¾ cup cornstarch

¾ cup tapioca starch

2 tsp. potato flour

½ tsp. cream of tartar

¼ tsp. baking soda

1 tsp. salt

COMBINE sugar, shortening, and margarine in mixer. In a small bowl, mix egg replacer and warm water thoroughly. Add egg replacer mixture and vanilla to sugar mixture and beat 1 minute. Add remaining ingredients and mix until well blended. Refrigerate dough for 1 hour. Grease an 8-inch round pan. Press dough into pan and bake at 350 degrees for 20–25 minutes. Frost with favorite cream cheese frosting (see p. 24). Cut up desired fruit into small pieces and put on top of frosted pizza. For a fun mini dessert, grease a cupcake tin, press dough into pan, and bake at 350 degrees for 10 minutes.

To make this recipe soy free: Substitute dairy-free margarine and shortening with an equal amount of soy-free margarine and shortening.

E   D   S   T   N   SH   F   W   G

desserts

Cream Cheese Frosting

Sometimes we need a cream cheese flavor. This works great on the dessert pizza.

1 (8-oz) tub dairy-free cream cheese
2 Tbsp. dairy-free margarine
1½ cups powdered sugar
1 tsp. vanilla (gluten free)

COMBINE ingredients in a bowl and beat well.

E   D   S   T   N   SH   F   W   G

Chocolate Drop Cookies

These are one of my son's favorite cookies, and they're super easy!

4 Tbsp. cocoa (dairy free)
½ cup soy milk
2 cups sugar
½ cup dairy-free margarine

½ cup soy nut butter
3 cups quick oats
1 tsp. vanilla (gluten free)

MIX cocoa, soy milk, sugar, and margarine together in saucepan, and boil for 1 minute. Remove from heat, add soy nut butter, quick oats, and vanilla, and mix until well blended. Spoon onto a sheet of plastic wrap and let cool before eating. Store in an airtight container. Makes 2 dozen.

To make this recipe gluten free: Substitute quick oats with an equal amount of gluten-free oats.

E   D   S   T   N   SH   F   W   G

Snickerdoodles

These cookies were a favorite when I would go to my grandmother's house. She always had plenty for her grandchilden, and they were yummy!

1 cup sugar
½ cup shortening
½ cup dairy-free margarine
3 tsp. egg replacer plus 4 Tbsp. warm water
½ Tbsp. vanilla (gluten free)
1 cup rice flour
¾ cup cornstarch
¾ cup tapioca starch
2 tsp. potato flour
½ tsp. cream of tartar
¼ tsp. baking soda
1 tsp. salt
½ cup sugar
½ tsp. cinnamon

COMBINE sugar, shortening, and margarine in mixer. In a small bowl, mix egg replacer and warm water thoroughly. Add egg replacer mixture and vanilla to sugar mixture, and mix 1 minute. Add remaining ingredients except sugar and cinnamon, and mix until well blended. Refrigerate dough for 1 hour. In a separate bowl mix sugar and cinnamon and set aside. Form dough into 1-inch balls, roll in cinnamon sugar, and place onto cookie sheet. Flatten with fork and bake at 350 degrees for 10–12 minutes. Let cool for 2 minutes before removing from cookie sheet. Makes 4½ dozen.

To make this recipe soy free: Substitute dairy-free margarine and shortening with an equal amount of soy-free margarine and shortening.

E   D   S   T   N   SH   F   W   G

Brownies

These are great when you need a quick chocolate treat. They are also great with chocolate frosting on top.

¾ cup dairy-free margarine
1¼ cups sugar
½ tsp. vanilla (gluten free)
¼ cup dairy-free chocolate chips
3 tsp. egg replacer plus 4 Tbsp. warm water
½ cup cocoa (dairy free)
1 cup rice flour
½ cup tapioca starch
½ tsp. salt
⅛ tsp. cream of tartar
1 tsp. baking soda

COMBINE margarine, sugar, and vanilla in mixer. In a small bowl, melt chocolate chips and add to margarine mixture. In another bowl, mix egg replacer and warm water thoroughly. Combine all ingredients and mix for 3 minutes. Press into an 8 x 8 pan, and bake at 350 degrees for 35 minutes. Let cool in pan before cutting into squares.

To make this recipe soy free: Substitute dairy-free margarine with an equal amount of soy-free margarine.

E   D   S   T   N   SH   F   W   G

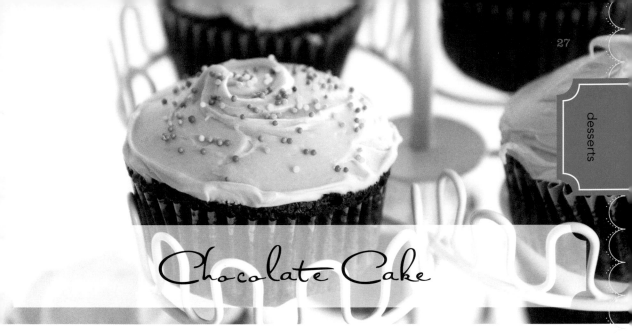

Chocolate Cake

I made the original version of this cake as a girl. It was a recipe from my great-grandmother, so I had to come up with an allergen-free one. Everyone loves it!

1¼ cups rice flour	2½ cups sugar
1 cup cornstarch	6 Tbsp. cocoa (dairy free)
1 cup tapioca starch	2 tsp. vanilla (gluten free)
2 tsp. potato flour	2 Tbsp. vinegar
2 tsp. baking soda	¾ cup oil
1 tsp. salt	2 cups water

IN a bowl, mix well by hand rice flour, cornstarch, tapioca starch, and potato flour. Mix in baking soda, salt, sugar, and cocoa. Make 3 wells in mixture and put vanilla in one, vinegar in the second, and oil in the third. Let sit for 2 minutes and then add water. Beat by hand until smooth. Pour mixture into greased 9 x 13 pan and bake at 350 degrees for 30–35 minutes. Allow to cool completely before frosting.

Tip: To make cupcakes, spoon mixture into lined cupcake pan and bake at 350 degrees for 18–20 minutes. These freeze well. Makes 28–30 cupcakes.

E   D   S   T   N   SH   F   W   G

Vanilla Cupcakes

I loved my chocolate cupcakes, but I wanted to try a vanilla one. My son now prefers the vanilla ones, but, of course, my daughter likes the chocolate. (What girl doesn't?) These freeze well too.

1¼ cups rice flour
1 cup cornstarch
1 cup plus 6 Tbsp. tapioca starch
2 tsp. potato flour
2 tsp. baking soda
1 tsp. salt
2½ cups sugar
2 tsp. vanilla (gluten free)
2 Tbsp. vinegar
¾ cup oil
2 cups water

IN a bowl, mix the following ingredients well by hand: rice flour, cornstarch, tapioca starch, and potato flour. Mix in baking soda, salt, and sugar. Make 3 wells in mixture and put vanilla in one, vinegar in the second, and oil in the third. Let sit for 2 minutes and then add water. Beat by hand until smooth. Spoon mixture into lined cupcake pan and bake at 350 degrees for 18–20 minutes. Allow to cool completely before frosting. Makes 28–30 cupcakes.

Tip: For a cake, pour batter into a greased 9 x 13 pan and bake at 350 degrees for 30–35 minutes.

E   D   S   T   N   SH   F   W   G

desserts

Fluffy Frosting

This frosting is just fun! It's thick so it looks great on any cake or cupcake, and it's super yummy!

¾ cup shortening

⅛ tsp. salt

1 tsp. vanilla (gluten free)

½ Tbsp. rice flour

3¾ cups powdered sugar

¼ cup water

MIX shortening, salt, and vanilla, until smooth. Add rice flour and beat for 2½ minutes. Add powdered sugar and beat 6 minutes. Add water and mix 2 minutes.

To make this recipe soy free: Substitute shortening with a soy-free shortening.

E   D   S   T   N   SH   F   W   G

Powdered Sugar Frosting

Here's a basic powdered sugar frosting that's allergen free, so it's worry free for birthdays!

¼ cup dairy-free margarine

⅓ cup powdered sugar

1 tsp. vanilla (gluten free)

⅔ cup powdered sugar

1 Tbsp. soy milk

MIX margarine, ⅓ cup powdered sugar, and vanilla until smooth. Then add ⅔ cup powdered sugar and soy milk and mix for 3 minutes until blended.

To make this recipe soy free: Substitute dairy-free margarine with an equal amount of soy-free margarine or shortening. Also substitute soy milk with an equal amount of rice or cow's milk.

E   D   S   T   N   SH   F   W   G

desserts

Chocolate Frosting

I love this chocolate frosting, I grew up with a cup of frosting and a spoon for a treat, so I had to create a special treat too.

2 Tbsp. dairy-free margarine	1 cup powdered sugar
¼ tsp. vanilla (gluten free)	2 Tbsp. cocoa (dairy free)
⅛ tsp. salt	1 Tbsp. soy milk

MIX all ingredients in a mixer until smooth, at least 3 minutes.

To make this recipe soy free: Substitute dairy-free margarine with an equal amount of soy-free margarine or shortening. Also substitute soy milk with an equal amount of rice or cow's milk.

E   D   S   T   N   SH   F   W   G

Caramel Sauce

This goes great on top of ice cream or alone for a little treat.

½ cup sugar
½ cup corn syrup
½ cup dairy-free creamer
2 Tbsp. dairy-free margarine
½ tsp. vanilla (gluten free)

IN a saucepan, combine sugar, corn syrup, and creamer, and bring to a boil. While stirring constantly, add margarine and vanilla. Cook until soft. Caramel sauce will thicken as it cools.

E   D   S   T   N   SH   F   W   G

Vanilla Ice Cream

Birthdays wouldn't be the same without ice cream, so be sure to make a batch or two for your next birthday party. Everyone will love it and ask for seconds. I find it is best the first day, but it hardly ever lasts in the house more than a day.

1 cup soy milk
¾ cup sugar
2 cups dairy-free creamer
1½ tsp. vanilla (gluten free)

IN a bowl, stir sugar into soy milk until sugar is dissolved, about 2 minutes. Stir in creamer and vanilla. Pour mixture into an ice cream maker, and follow your ice cream maker's instructions. Store uneaten ice cream in an airtight container in freezer. Lasts up to 1 week.

E   D   S   T   N   SH   F   W   G

Sweetened Condensed Milk

I needed to come up with a sweetened condensed milk so I could make one of my favorite recipes—the cookie bars. I did it!

¼ cup water
½ cup sugar
1 Tbsp. dairy-free margarine
1 cup soy milk powder

COMBINE water and sugar in a saucepan, and heat until sugar dissolves. Pour sugar mixture into a blender. Add margarine and blend. Gradually add soy milk powder, while blending, until smooth.

E   D   S   T   N   SH   F   W   G

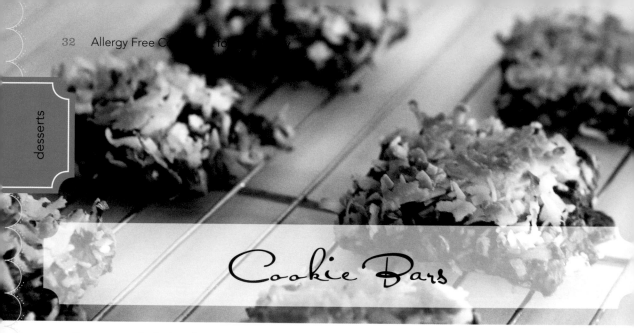

Cookie Bars

I was so excited when I came up with the recipe for the sweetened condensed milk so I could make these cookie bars. I get lots of requests to make these for family dinners.

¼ cup dairy-free margarine
¾ cup graham crackers (see p. 38)
1 batch of sweetened condensed milk (see p. 31)
¾ cup dairy-free chocolate chips
½ cup coconut flakes*

MELT margarine and pour into an 8 x 8 pan. Crush graham crackers and spread in pan evenly. Pour sweetened condensed milk over crackers. Sprinkle chocolate chips and coconut flakes on top. Bake at 350 degrees for 25–30 minutes. Let cool completely and cut into squares.

* If you suffer from a tree nut allergy, you may need to avoid coconut. If so, just leave coconut out of the recipe!

E   D   S   T   N   SH   F   W   G

Fudge

I grew up making fudge at Christmastime and wanted my family to enjoy this wonderful treat.

¼ cup sugar

¼ cup brown sugar

½ Tbsp. cocoa (dairy free)

1 Tbsp. corn syrup

2 Tbsp. soy milk

¼ cup soy nut butter

½ Tbsp. dairy-free margarine

¼ tsp. vanilla (gluten free)

MIX sugars, cocoa, corn syrup, and soy milk in saucepan and bring to a boil. Add soy nut butter, margarine, and vanilla. Stir constantly to prevent burning. Pour into a greased 9 x 13 pan and let set. Cut into squares.

E   D   S   T   N   SH   F   W   G

desserts

Chocolate Soy Nut Butter Balls

My husband grew up eating these treats every Christmas, thanks to his grandmother. So, through many attempts, here is my version of his grandmother's treat, and we think they're great!

¼ cup dairy-free margarine
⅓ cup soy nut butter
1 cup powdered sugar
½ cup dairy-free chocolate chips

MIX margarine, soy nut butter, and powdered sugar until smooth. Place mixture in fridge for 10 minutes. Form margarine mixture into small 1-inch balls. Melt chocolate. Dip balls into melted chocolate and freeze for 10 minutes. Store in freezer. Makes 16–18 balls.

E   D   S   T   N   SH   F   W   G

Pie Crust

I really enjoy eating pies and had to come up with a pie crust recipe.

1 cup rice flour
1 cup tapioca starch
1 tsp. salt
1 cup shortening
¼ cup cold water

COMBINE all ingredients in a bowl and mix well. Form into a ball and roll dough into a circular shape onto a rice-floured surface. Place rolled dough into a pie pan. Bake at 350 degrees for 10–15 minutes. To finsh pie, add your favorite allergy-free filling and bake as directed. Makes one crust.

To make this recipe soy free: Substitute shortening with a soy-free shortening.

E   D   S   T   N   SH   F   W   G

Apple Pie Filling

Here is a great pie filling for the pie crust recipe. It is so easy and tastes great for the holidays or for any occasion.

4–5 apples (peeled and sliced)
2 Tbsp. lemon juice
3 Tbsp. rice flour
½ tsp. cinnamon
¼ tsp. nutmeg
1 cup sugar
¼ cup brown sugar
3 Tbsp. dairy-free margarine
dash of salt

PLACE apples in a bowl. Pour lemon juice over apples. Add rice flour, cinnamon, nutmeg, sugars, margarine, and salt. Mix well. Pour in pie shell. Bake at 400 degrees for 1 hour.

To make this recipe soy free: Substitute dairy-free margarine with an equal amount of soy-free margarine or shortening.

E   D   S   T   N   SH   F   W   G

Apple Crisp

One of my favorite desserts growing up was my mom's apple crisp. I wanted my kids to enjoy it too. It is especially good in the fall and winter months.

4 cups apples, peeled and sliced
¼ cup orange juice or lemon juice
1 cup sugar
¾ cup rice flour
½ tsp. cinnamon
¼ tsp. nutmeg
½ cup dairy-free margarine
dash of salt

PLACE apples in a greased pie pan. Pour orange juice or lemon juice over apples. In a bowl, mix together sugar, rice flour, cinnamon, nutmeg, margarine, and salt. Sprinkle on top of apples. Bake at 375 degrees for 45 minutes or until apples are tender and topping is crisp.

To make this recipe soy free: Substitute dairy-free margarine with an equal amount of soy-free margarine.

E   D   S   T   N   SH   F   W   G

Graham Crackers

I loved making graham cracker houses at Christmastime. This graham cracker recipe allows my kids to continue the tradition.

½ cup dairy-free margarine
1 cup brown sugar
2 Tbsp. honey
½ tsp. egg replacer plus 2 Tbsp. warm water
1 cup rice flour
¾ cup tapioca starch
1 tsp. potato flour
¼ tsp. cream of tartar
⅛ tsp. baking soda
½ tsp. salt

MIX margarine, brown sugar, and honey until smooth. In a small bowl, thoroughly mix egg replacer with warm water and add to sugar mixture. Add remaining ingredients and mix for 3 minutes. Roll dough ¼-inch thick onto rice-floured surface, and cut into desired shapes. Bake at 350 degrees for 10–12 minutes. Let cool for 3 minutes before removing from cookie sheet.

To make this recipe soy free: Substitute dairy-free margarine with an equal amount of soy-free margarine.

E   D   S   T   N   SH   F   W   G

Graham Cracker Crust

After I made up the graham cracker recipe, I thought "Wow! Now I can do a graham cracker crust and make some pies."

1½ cups graham crackers, crushed (see p. 38)
2 Tbsp. sugar
2 Tbsp. dairy-free margarine, melted

IN a bowl mix crushed graham crackers, sugar, and margarine. Press into a 9-inch pie pan. Bake at 350 degrees 10–12 minutes until golden.

To make this recipe soy free: Substitute dairy-free margarine with an equal amount of soy-free margarine.

E   D   S   T   N   SH   F   W   G

Cream Cheese Dessert

I love cheesecake. Here is my allergen-free version of cheesecake. I could eat the whole pie by myself!

4 cups marshmallows (gluten and egg free)
⅓ cup soy milk
2 cups dairy-free creamer
¼ cup sugar

2 (8-oz. pkgs.) packages dairy-free cream cheese
½ cup sugar
1 graham cracker crust (see above)

HEAT marshmallows and soy milk on stove until melted. While waiting, beat creamer and ¼ cup sugar for 3 minutes. Add cream cheese and ½ cup sugar, and beat until smooth. Add marshmallow mixture and mix well. Pour into a graham cracker crust and place in freezer until set.

E   D   S   T   N   SH   F   W   G

desserts

Raspberry Pie

I was so happy when I came up with the graham cracker crust because I could then make one of my favorite childhood pies. When I go to family functions, my niece always wants me to bring my raspberry or strawberry pie. She says it's her favorite pie ever.

1 cup sugar
1 cup cold water
3 Tbsp. cornstarch
3 Tbsp. raspberry gelatin (dry)
4 cups raspberries, fresh or frozen
1 graham cracker crust (see p. 39)

MIX sugar, water, and cornstarch well. Cook in microwave for 4 minutes or on stove, stirring constantly until mixture begins to boil. Add gelatin and stir. Let cool. Place berries in crust. When gelatin mixture is cool, pour over raspberries in crust. Let set in fridge for 1 hour.

VARIATION: Substitute strawberries for raspberries and strawberry gelatin for raspberry gelatin.

E   D   S   T   N   SH   F   W   G

Donuts

My family enjoys making these treats together.

½ cup rice flour

¼ cup tapioca starch

¼ cup cornstarch

1 tsp. potato flour

1 Tbsp. sugar

1 tsp. xanthan gum

½ tsp. cream of tartar

¼ tsp. baking soda

½ tsp. salt

2 Tbsp. oil

½ cup plus 1–2 Tbsp. cold water

1 cup oil, for pan

MIX all ingredients except 1 cup oil in a bowl until well blended. Roll dough on rice-floured surface and cut into circles. Add oil to frying pan and heat. When ready, drop circles of dough one by one into hot oil and fry 2–3 minutes on each side. Lay donuts on a paper towel to cool.

E   D   S   T   N   SH   F   W   G

Donut Glaze

1¼ cups powdered sugar

½ tsp. vanilla (gluten free)

¼ cup cold water

¼ cup dairy-free margarine

MIX ingredients in a mixer until smooth. Pour over donuts.

To make this recipe soy free: Substitute dairy-free margarine with an equal amount of soy-free margarine.

E   D   S   T   N   SH   F   W   G

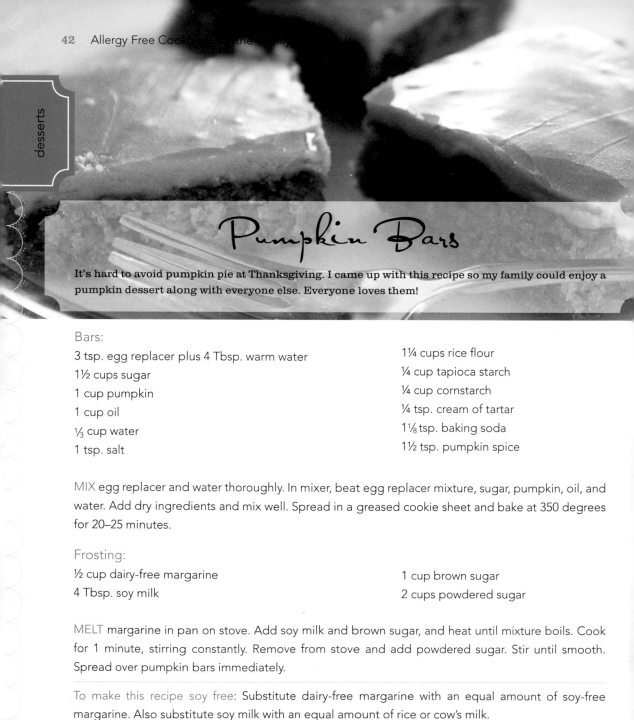

Pumpkin Bars

It's hard to avoid pumpkin pie at Thanksgiving. I came up with this recipe so my family could enjoy a pumpkin dessert along with everyone else. Everyone loves them!

Bars:

3 tsp. egg replacer plus 4 Tbsp. warm water

1½ cups sugar

1 cup pumpkin

1 cup oil

⅓ cup water

1 tsp. salt

1¼ cups rice flour

¼ cup tapioca starch

¼ cup cornstarch

¼ tsp. cream of tartar

1⅛ tsp. baking soda

1½ tsp. pumpkin spice

MIX egg replacer and water thoroughly. In mixer, beat egg replacer mixture, sugar, pumpkin, oil, and water. Add dry ingredients and mix well. Spread in a greased cookie sheet and bake at 350 degrees for 20–25 minutes.

Frosting:

½ cup dairy-free margarine

4 Tbsp. soy milk

1 cup brown sugar

2 cups powdered sugar

MELT margarine in pan on stove. Add soy milk and brown sugar, and heat until mixture boils. Cook for 1 minute, stirring constantly. Remove from stove and add powdered sugar. Stir until smooth. Spread over pumpkin bars immediately.

To make this recipe soy free: Substitute dairy-free margarine with an equal amount of soy-free margarine. Also substitute soy milk with an equal amount of rice or cow's milk.

E   D   S   T   N   SH   F   W   G

Drinks

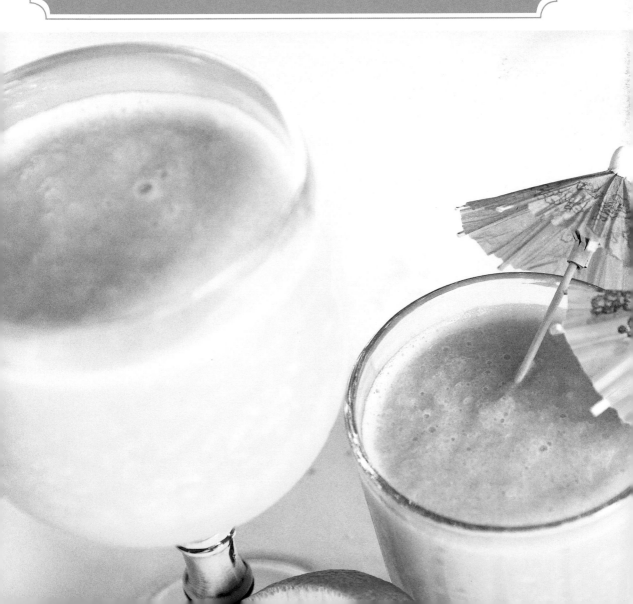

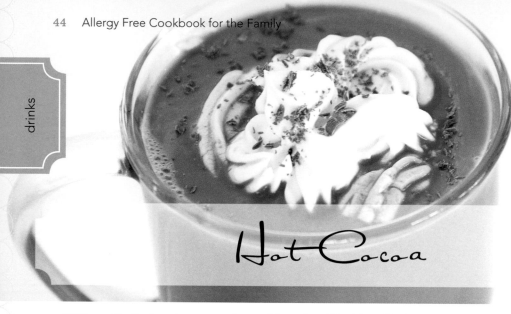

Hot Cocoa

This was the first recipe my son learned to make all by himself using the microwave. He was so proud of himself and so was I!

1½ tsp. cocoa (dairy free)
2 Tbsp. sugar
1 cup soy milk

COMBINE ingredients into pan on stove. Heat on medium, and stir for 1 minute. Continue stirring occasionally for 5 minutes until warm.

TO MAKE this treat in the microwave, pour milk into a microwave safe mug, and heat for 1 minute. Add remaining ingredients, and stir until smooth. Enjoy!

Tip: You can garnish with a dairy-free whipped topping and dairy-free chocolate shavings.
To make this recipe soy free: Substitute soy milk with an equal amount of rice or cow's milk.

E   D   S   T   N   SH   F   W   G

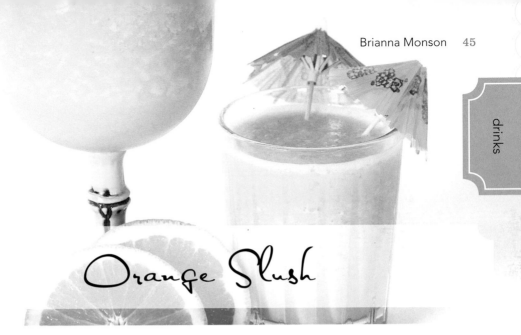

Orange Slush

This slush is so easy and is great with any breakfast. My family loves it with waffles.

1 (12-oz.) can orange juice (concentrate)
1 cup soy milk
1 cup cold water
½ cup sugar
2 tsp. vanilla (gluten free)
12–15 ice cubes

COMBINE ingredients in a blender. Mix until smooth and serve.

To make this recipe soy free: Substitute soy milk with an equal amount of rice or cow's milk.

E   D   S   T   N   SH   F   W   G

Peach Smoothie

We love this smoothie in the summer when peaches are ripe. I freeze peaches so we can have this treat year round.

4 cups frozen peaches (slightly thawed)
¼ cup sugar
½ cup soy milk

COMBINE ingredients in a blender. Mix until smooth and serve.

Tip. To make this drink slushy, just add 12 ice cubes.
To make this recipe soy free: Substitute soy milk with an equal amount of rice or cow's milk.

E   D   S   T   N   SH   F   W   G

Frozen Strawberry Smoothie

This smoothie is great with breakfast or as a summertime treat.

2 cups frozen strawberries
1 cup soy milk
1 Tbsp. sugar

COMBINE ingredients in a blender. Mix until smooth and serve.

To make this recipe soy free: Substitute soy milk with an equal amount of rice or cow's milk.

E   D   S   T   N   SH   F   W   G

Fresh Strawberry Smoothie

My kids love this smoothie because it isn't too cold!

2 cups fresh strawberries
½ cup soy milk
¼ cup sugar
10–12 ice cubes

COMBINE all ingredients in a blender. Mix until smooth and serve.

To make this recipe soy free: **Substitute soy milk with an equal amount of rice or cow's milk.**

E   D   S   T   N   SH   F   W   G

drinks

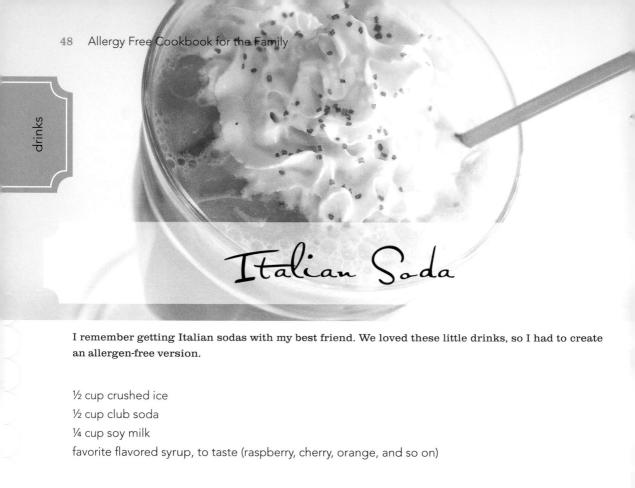

Italian Soda

I remember getting Italian sodas with my best friend. We loved these little drinks, so I had to create an allergen-free version.

½ cup crushed ice
½ cup club soda
¼ cup soy milk
favorite flavored syrup, to taste (raspberry, cherry, orange, and so on)

FILL cup with crushed ice. Add club soda and soy milk and stir. Add flavoring to taste, stir, and enjoy!

To make this recipe soy free: Substitute soy milk with an equal amount of rice or cow's milk.

E   D   S   T   N   SH   F   W   G

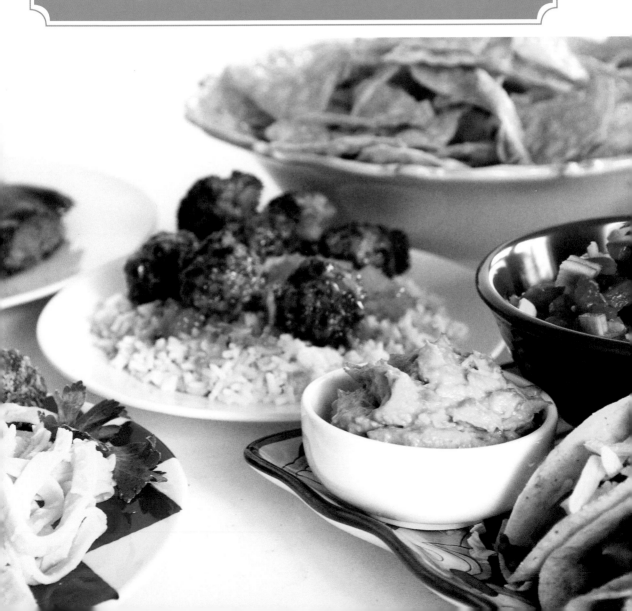

Main Dishes

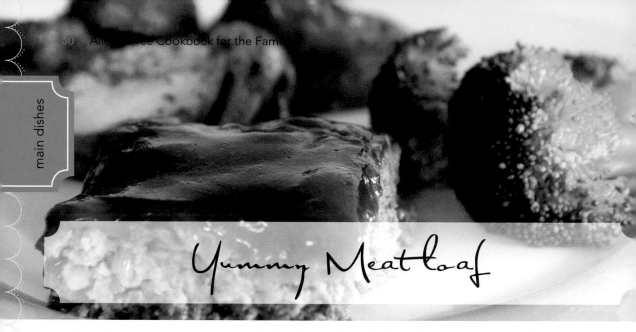

Yummy Meatloaf

The original recipe has been a family favorite, and I couldn't go without it. So I tailored it to meet the needs of my family. Those that eat it and know the original love this even better. Those that try it for the first time want seconds every time.

2½ pounds hamburger
½ cup onion, chopped
1½ cups quick oats
1 cup soy milk
1½ tsp. salt
¼ tsp. pepper
½ cup grated carrots
2 Tbsp. oil
½ cup brown sugar

Topping:
⅓ cup ketchup
4 Tbsp. brown sugar
2 Tbsp. mustard
1 tsp. honey

HEAT oven to 350 degrees. Mix meatloaf ingredients in a bowl. Place in a greased 9 x 13 pan. Mix topping ingredients and spread over meatloaf. Bake for 1–1½ hours.

To make this recipe gluten free: Substitute quick oats with an equal amount of gluten-free oats.
To make this recipe soy free: Substitute soy milk with an equal amount of rice or cow's milk.

E   D   S   T   N   SH   F   W   G

Meatballs

These freeze very well! They're perfect for making quick meals.

1 lb. hamburger
1 cup quick oats
1½ Tbsp. oil
1 tsp. salt
⅛ tsp. pepper
1 Tbsp. parsley
2 Tbsp. oil, for pan

MIX all ingredients except oil and form into balls. Heat skillet with 2 tablespoons oil. Cook meatballs in skillet until brown. Serve plain or with rice. Makes 15–17 1-inch balls.

Tip: Freeze on a cookie sheet first and then put in a freezer bag to store. Then you can simply take out the amount you need.

To make this recipe gluten free: Substitute quick oats with an equal amount of gluten-free oats.

E   D   S   T   N   SH   F   W   G

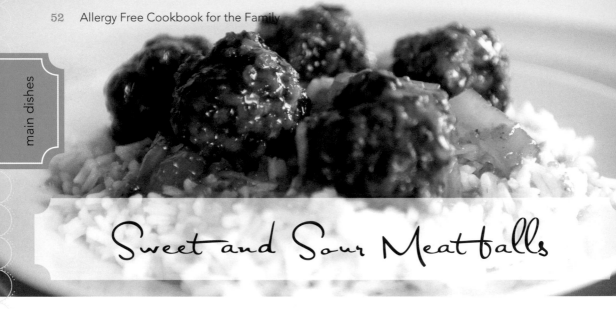

Sweet and Sour Meatballs

My kids love this sweet and sour sauce on their meatballs, and it's super easy to make. If you've premade your meatballs and frozen them, you'll have a great dinner in no time.

Sweet and Sour Sauce:

2 Tbsp. cornstarch

1½ cups brown sugar

1 (20-oz.) can pineapple chunks

1/3 cup vinegar

1 Tbsp. soy sauce (gluten free)

PREPARE meatballs from p. 51.

HEAT cornstarch, brown sugar, and juice from canned pineapple on stove. Add the pineapple chunks, vinegar, and soy sauce. Simmer for 10 minutes, stirring frequently. Pour over meatballs and serve.

E   D   S   T   N   SH   F   W   G

Porcupine Meatballs

When I was a young girl, this was the first main dish I made all by myself, but the recipe called for tomato soup as its base. It's much easier with a can of soup, but I created this for the allergen-free version.

1 lb. hamburger
½ cup rice, cooked
¼ cup onion, chopped
1 tsp. salt
¼ tsp. pepper
2 Tbsp. oil
1 (14.5-oz.) can tomato sauce
1 Tbsp. sugar
½ tsp. chili powder (optional)
½ cup water

MIX hamburger, rice, onion, salt, and pepper together. Form into meatballs. Heat oil in skillet. Cook meatballs in skillet until done. Add tomato sauce, sugar, chili powder, and water to meatballs and bring to a boil. Simmer for 20 minutes.

E   D   S   T   N   SH   F   W   G

Sloppy Joes

This is a great recipe to make for large groups. We enjoy having these at our family reunions. They are easy to make, and everyone loves them.

1 lb. hamburger
½ onion, chopped
1¼ cups ketchup
½ cup water
1 Tbsp. vinegar
1 Tbsp. brown sugar
½ tsp. salt
½ tsp. mustard
½ tsp. chili powder (optional)

BROWN hamburger in skillet. Mix in remaining ingredients and simmer for 10 minutes. Scoop mixture onto your favorite toasted bread.

Corn Dog Bites

This recipe took a lot of trial and error. I finally added a little guar gum, which I had never heard of before, and it worked. The kids love these!

10 hot dogs (dairy and gluten free)
3 tsp. egg replacer plus 4 Tbsp. warm water
1 cup corn meal
2 cups masa flour
⅔ cup honey
1 tsp. mustard
2 tsp. cream of tartar
1 tsp. baking soda
4 Tbsp. oil
2 cups water
2 tsp. guar gum
¾ cup oil, for skillet

RINSE hot dogs and set aside. In a bowl mix egg replacer and warm water thoroughly. Add all other ingredients and mix well. Cut each hot dog into 3 pieces and form mixture around them (mixture will be sticky). Heat a skillet with oil and fry corn dogs until golden.

E   D   S   T   N   SH   F   W   G

Chicken Casserole

I remember eating this as a child—my mom made it with cream of mushroom soup. So here is my version, and it's creamy without the can!

2 cups rice, cooked
3 cups broccoli, cooked and chopped
2 cups cubed chicken, cooked
½ cup onion, chopped
½ tsp. garlic powder
1 Tbsp. dairy-free margarine

Sauce:
¾ cup dairy-free margarine
¼ cup cornstarch
¼ cup tapioca starch
¼ cup rice flour
½ tsp. potato flour
3 cups soy milk
1½ tsp. salt
pepper, to taste

AFTER cooking rice, broccoli, and chicken, set aside. In a frying pan, sauté onion and garlic powder in margarine. Mix in cooked rice, broccoli, and chicken. In a saucepan, stir in sauce ingredients. Heat on medium, stirring until thickened. Put broccoli mixture in a 9 x 13 pan, and pour sauce over the top. Bake in oven at 350 degrees for 20 minutes.

To make this recipe soy free: Substitute dairy-free margarine with an equal amount of soy-free margarine. Also substitute soy milk with an equal amount of rice or cow's milk.

E   D   S   T   N   SH   F   W   G

Tater Tot™ Casserole

My kids ask for this dinner because they love tater tots, and I love it because they get their vegetables too!

1 lb. hamburger
¾ cup dairy-free margarine
¼ cup cornstarch
¼ cup tapioca starch
¼ cup rice flour
½ tsp. potato flour
1¾ cups soy milk
½ tsp. salt
pepper, to taste
1 (15-oz.) can corn, drained
15–20 tater tots (dairy and gluten free)

COOK hamburger. While cooking, place margarine, cornstarch, tapioca starch, flours, soy milk, salt, and pepper in saucepan. Heat and stir until smooth. In a 9 x 13 pan, mix sauce, hamburger, and corn. Place tater tots™ on top of mixture, and bake in the oven at 350 degrees for 18–20 minutes.

Tip: You can substitute the corn for any other vegetable of your choice.
To make this recipe soy free: Substitute dairy-free margarine with an equal amount of soy-free margarine. Also substitute soy milk with an equal amount of rice or cow's milk.

E   D   S   T   N   SH   F   W   G

Easy Pork Chops

This is great for a night when you don't have a lot of time to cook.

1 cup corn cereal (gluten free)
½ tsp. salt
⅛ tsp. pepper
½ Tbsp. parsley
1 cup soy milk
1 lb. pork chops

IN a bowl, crush corn cereal. Add salt, pepper, and parsley, and mix well. Pour soy milk into another bowl. Dip pork chops one by one into soy milk and then coat in cereal mixture. Spray pan with gluten- and dairy-free cooking spray. Heat frying pan, and fry pork chops until done.

VARIATION: Use chicken in place of pork chops.
To make this recipe soy free: Substitute soy milk with an equal amount of rice or cow's milk.

E   D   S   T   N   SH   F   W   G

Round Steak Dish

My mom made this meal often when I was young. I adapted it, and you can't tell the difference. I double the recipe because everyone loves it so much. Just after creating this to fit with our allergen needs, I had my in-laws in town and made this for dinner. They loved it and asked for seconds, so be sure to make plenty!

4 servings of cooked rice
1 lb. round steak
1 Tbsp. oil
1 Tbsp. paprika
1 tsp. minced garlic
1¾ cups water
1 cup onion, chopped
2 Tbsp. cornstarch
⅓ cup soy sauce (gluten free)

PREPARE rice and set aside. Cut meat into thin strips. Heat oil on medium in frying pan. Brown meat. Sprinkle paprika over meat. Add garlic and 1½ cups water. Simmer, covered, for 30 minutes. Stir in onions. Cover and cook 5 minutes. Add cornstarch, ¼ cup water, and soy sauce. Cook and stir until thick. Serve over rice.

E   D   S   T   N   SH   F   W   G

Cornbread Bake

This is a fun dish to serve for any occasion.

1 lb. hamburger
½ cup onion, chopped
1 Tbsp. oil
2 tsp. chili powder (optional)
¾ tsp. salt
1 (14.5-oz.) can stewed tomatoes
1 (16-oz.) can kidney beans
cornbread batter (cornbread recipe on p. 9)

BROWN hamburger and onion in oil. Add seasonings and tomatoes. Simmer for 15 minutes. Add beans and simmer for 3 more minutes. Pour mixture into a 2-quart baking dish. Top with cornbread batter and bake at 350 degrees for 20 minutes.

E   D   S   T   N   SH   F   W   G

Enchilada Casserole

My kids love to help with this meal because they get to be in charge of layering the ingredients.

1 lb. hamburger
1 onion, chopped
1 (15-oz.) can corn, drained
1 (14.5-oz.) can tomato sauce
2 Tbsp. sugar
2 tsp. chili powder (optional)
½ cup olives, sliced
3–4 corn tortillas

BROWN hamburger and onion. Add corn, tomato sauce, sugar, chili powder, and olives, and simmer for 10 minutes. In a 2-quart baking dish, alternate corn tortillas and then sauce, 3 to 4 layers deep. Bake at 350 degrees for 20 minutes.

Tip: If you love a dairy-free cheese, try adding it on top and cooking it until melted.

E   D   S   T   N   SH   F   W   G

Fried Chicken

This is an easy recipe for fried chicken, and the kids will love it.

2 cups rice flour
1 tsp. salt
½ tsp. pepper

2 Tbsp. oil
8 chicken pieces

MIX rice flour, salt, and pepper in bowl. Put oil in pan and heat on medium. Dip chicken in flour mixture, and then place in hot pan and fry for 8 minutes on each side.

Tip: May also bake in oven at 350 degrees for 1 hour.

E   D   S   T   N   SH   F   W   G

Apricot Chicken

This recipe was created through experimenting with a jar of apricot jam. I think you'll love the results as much as my family does.

6 boneless chicken breasts
1 jar apricot jam
½ onion, chopped
2 Tbsp. dairy-free margarine
1 cup chicken broth (gluten free)

PLACE chicken breasts in a slow cooker. Add 1 jar of apricot jam. Sauté onion in margarine in frying pan, add chicken broth, and stir. Pour onion mixture in slow cooker, and stir. Cook on low 4–6 hours.

To make this recipe soy free: Substitute dairy-free margarine with an equal amount of soy-free margarine.

E   D   S   T   N   SH   F   W   G

Shepherd's Pie

My mom made this recipe with tomato soup when I was young. This is a twist on the traditional recipe without the tomato soup.

main dishes

1 lb. hamburger
1 (14.5-oz.) can stewed tomatoes
1 Tbsp. sugar
1 (14.5-oz) can green beans
½ tsp. salt
8 servings mashed potatoes, prepared
   (recipe on p. 80)

BROWN hamburger. Combine meat, tomatoes, sugar, beans, and salt in a 9 x 13 pan. Prepare mashed potatoes and spread on top of meat mixture. Bake at 350 degrees for 30 minutes.

E   D   S   T   N   SH   F   W   G

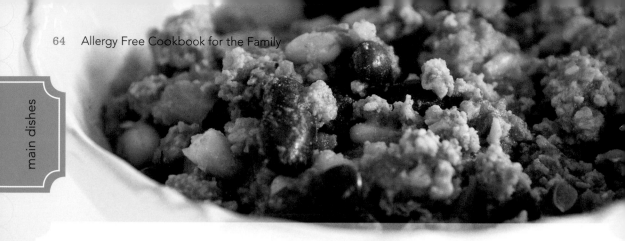

main dishes

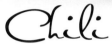

It is hard to find chili that is allergen free, so I created this recipe. My family loves to have it on a cold rainy day. I also use it to make Coney Dogs.

1 lb. hamburger
1 small onion, chopped
1 can diced tomatoes, optional
1 (15-oz.) can great northern beans, drained
1 (15-oz.) can red beans, drained
1–2 cups water
1½ tsp. salt
¼ tsp. pepper
½ tsp. garlic powder
½ tsp. oregano
½ tsp. basil

BROWN hamburger with onion. Combine all ingredients in a pot and simmer for 20 minutes, stirring occasionally.

Tip: This also freezes well. You may also substitute the beans for another bean of your choice.

E   D   S   T   N   SH   F   W   G

Fajitas

This is probably my husband's favorite dish, and I love when he makes it!

4 Tbsp. dairy-free margarine
½ onion, chopped
½ red pepper, chopped
½ green pepper, chopped
1 lb. beef or chicken, cut in strips
½ Tbsp. salt
¼ tsp. pepper
minced garlic, to taste
8–10 corn tortillas

MELT 2 tablespoons margarine on stove. Add onion and peppers, and cook until tender. In another pan melt 2 tablespoons margarine, and add cut up meat. Cook until meat is done. Add meat to vegetables, and add salt, pepper, and garlic. Simmer for 5 minutes. Place ingredients inside tortilla, and serve!

To make this recipe soy free: Substitute dairy-free margarine with an equal amount of soy-free margarine.

E   D   S   T   N   SH   F   W   G

Cabbage Casserole

My mom made fantastic cabbage rolls when I was growing up. Here is my creation that doesn't have to be rolled, so it's much easier.

1 lb. hamburger
1¼ cups water
1 (6-oz.) can tomato paste
3 Tbsp. sugar
½ tsp. salt
¼ cup soy milk
1 head of cabbage, cut up in small pieces

BROWN hamburger. Add water, tomato paste, sugar, salt, and soy milk, and simmer for 10 minutes. In a 9 x 13 pan, place a layer of washed cabbage. Then spoon tomato mixture on top. Continue to alternate cabbage and tomato mixture. Bake at 350 degrees for 30 minutes.

To make this recipe soy free: Substitute soy milk with an equal amount of rice or cow's milk.

E   D   S   T   N   SH   F   W   G

Pumpkin Surprise

This has become a family tradition. I make this every Halloween, and the kids love it.

1 medium pumpkin
1 lb. hamburger
1 cup onion, chopped
1 cup green pepper, chopped
2 cups rice
2 cups water
1 cup chicken or beef broth (gluten free)

CLEAN out a pumpkin and bake at 350 degrees for 25 minutes. Brown hamburger, onion, and green pepper. Add rice, water, and broth. Simmer, covered, for 20 minutes. Put mixture in pumpkin, and bake at 350 degrees for 30–45 minutes.

E   D   S   T   N   SH   F   W   G

Tacos

Our family has tacos once a week, and everyone pitches in with the preparation. I love the help!

½ lb. hamburger
1 (16-oz.) can refried beans
2 Tbsp. oil (to put in pan if you fry your shells)
8 corn taco shells

Toppings: ketchup, lettuce, tomatoes, olives, onions, avocados, or corn

COOK hamburger in a pan. In another pan, warm refried beans. Prepare desired toppings and place in individual bowls. Place taco shells on a cookie sheet and broil for 3 minutes or fry in a pan on medium heat. Let everyone spoon favorite ingredients into taco shells.

Tip: We make the salsa on p. 85 to go with our tacos.

E   D   S   T   N   SH   F   W   G

Spaghetti and Sauce

I have found that many store-bought spaghetti sauces are not suitable for the allergy sufferer, so I created this sauce to take its place.

Sauce:

1 lb. hamburger

½ onion, chopped

1 (8-oz.) can tomato sauce

1 tsp. sugar

2 tsp. garlic salt

¼ tsp. chili powder

½ tsp. salt

⅛ tsp. pepper

Noodles:

1 package of your favorite noodles (gluten & egg free)

8 cups water

1 tsp. salt

BROWN hamburger and onion together. Mix together all the sauce ingredients. Simmer for 10 minutes. While sauce is cooking, fix spaghetti noodles according to package directions. Combine noodles, sauce, and meat together and serve.

E   D   S   T   N   SH   F   W   G

White Sauce

Use this recipe to substitute for cream of chicken or mushroom soup, and you'll be happy!

¼ cup cornstarch
¼ cup tapioca starch
¼ cup rice flour
½ tsp. potato flour
¼ cup dairy-free margarine
1¾ cups soy milk
½ tsp. salt
pepper, to taste

MIX cornstarch, tapioca starch, rice flour, and potato flour, and set aside. In a saucepan, melt margarine. When melted, add soy milk and stir until blended. Add ¼ cup of the flour mixture and stir. Add salt and pepper to taste. Store leftover flour mixture in an airtight container for future recipes.

Tip: Add chicken or mushrooms, if desired.
To make this recipe soy free: Substitute dairy-free margarine with an equal amount of soy-free margarine. Also substitute soy milk with an equal amount of rice or cow's milk.

E   D   S   T   N   SH   F   W   G

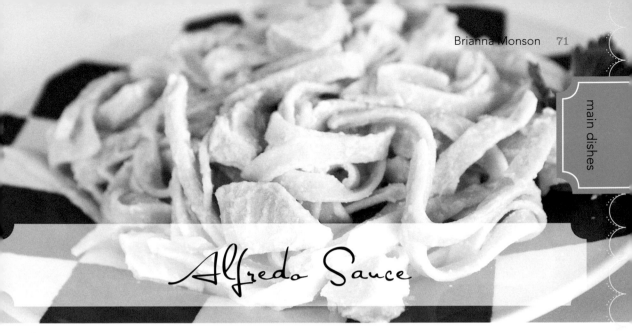

Alfredo Sauce

This recipe took some trial and error, but it was worth it!

5 Tbsp. dairy-free cream cheese
½ cup dairy-free margarine
2 cups dairy-free creamer
1 tsp. garlic powder

IN a mixer blend cream cheese with margarine and creamer. Pour into a saucepan, and heat until bubbly. Add garlic powder and stir for 1 minute. Pour over your favorite cooked noodles. Let sauce sit to thicken.

Tip: You can add cooked chicken or broccoli.

E   D   S   T   N   SH   F   W   G

Italian Chicken

I created this as an easy slow cooker dish and love to make it when we have company. I also take my slow cooker and the ingredients when I go on trips because it's so easy to make.

4–6 boneless skinless chicken breasts
½ bottle of Italian salad dressing (gluten, egg, and dairy free)
4 cups rice

PLACE chicken into a slow cooker. Pour dressing over chicken and cook on low for 4–6 hours. Prepare rice just before serving. Serve chicken over rice.

E   D   S   T   N   SH   F   W   G

Honey Ham

We love to have this for the holidays.

1 ham, 10-15 pounds
¼ cup honey
¼ cup brown sugar
1 (20-oz.) can crushed pineapple

PLACE ham into a slow cooker. Put honey, brown sugar, and pineapple over the top. Cook on low for 4–6 hours.

E   D   S   T   N   SH   F   W   G

Shish Kebabs

These are fun to make. Your kids can help with this meal, so enjoy the family time.

1 lb. chicken or beef, cubed
1 (20-oz.) can chunk pineapple
1 cup onion, cut in pieces
1 cup potato, cut in pieces
1 cup green pepper, cut in pieces
10 skewers

PUT items onto skewers, alternating each food. Leave small space between each piece to allow cooking. Bake at 350 degrees for 15–20 minutes or grill on barbeque for 4–7 minutes, rotating.

E   D   S   T   N   SH   F   W   G

Foil Bake

My husband makes these for camping trips, so I adjusted it to have anytime—camping or at home.

1 lb. hamburger   ½ tsp. salt
4 potatoes, cubed   ¼ tsp. pepper
3–4 carrots, sliced   4–6 foil sheets
1 onion, sliced

BROWN hamburger. Tear off 4–6 sheets of foil about 1-foot by 1-foot. Place hamburger, potatoes, carrots, onion, salt, and pepper in each foil sheet. Fold in each side and wrap. Bake at 375 degrees for 40 minutes.

E   D   S   T   N   SH   F   W   G

Cabbage Skillet

I created this recipe by using some leftovers in the fridge, and now it is a dish I make on purpose! It is so quick and easy, and the kids love it.

1 lb. hamburger
½ cup red onion, chopped
1 (10-oz.) package coleslaw mix or 8 cups cabbage, cut up
1 tsp. salt
¼ tsp. chili powder
⅛ tsp. sesame seed oil (optional)

IN a skillet, brown hamburger and onion. Add coleslaw package or cabbage and stir. Add salt, chili powder, and sesame seed oil. Cook on medium, covered for 5 minutes. Serve.

Side Dishes

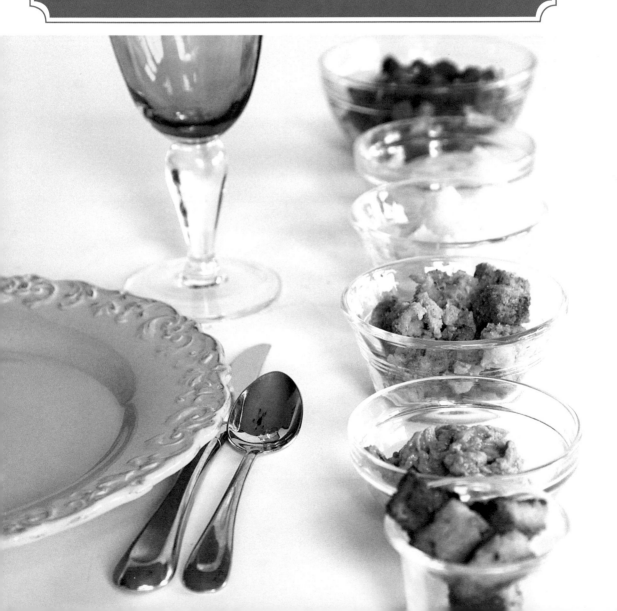

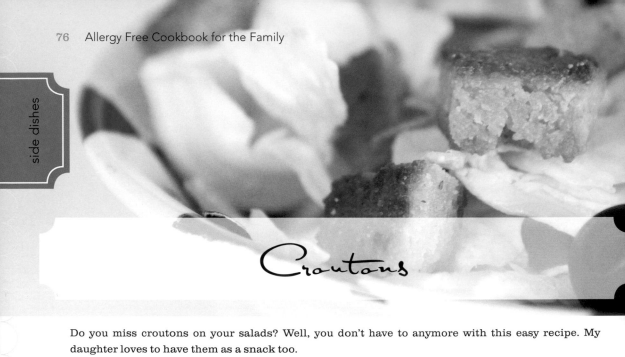

Croutons

Do you miss croutons on your salads? Well, you don't have to anymore with this easy recipe. My daughter loves to have them as a snack too.

1½ cups bread, cubed (I use the Bread Machine Sandwich Bread recipe p. 5)
¼ cup dairy-free margarine, melted
¼ tsp. salt
pinch of pepper
⅛ tsp. garlic powder
¼ tsp. parsley flakes

MELT margarine and stir in salt, pepper, garlic powder, and parsley flakes. Dip bread into margarine mixture, and place on a cookie sheet. Broil 3–4 minutes on each side.

To make this recipe soy free: Substitute dairy-free margarine with an equal amount of soy-free margarine.

E   D   S   T   N   SH   F   W   G

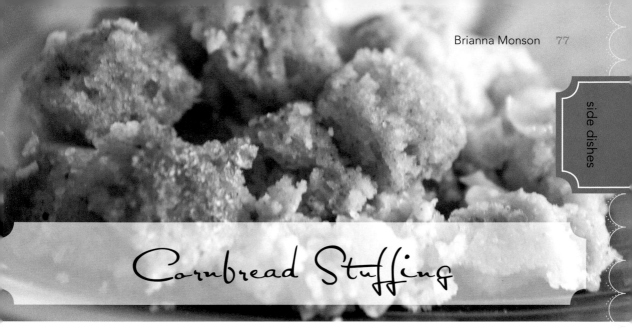

Cornbread Stuffing

I love stuffing at Thanksgiving, but of course the traditional stuffing is not safe. So I created this cornbread stuffing and take it to our family Thanksgivings. Everyone asks for it each year.

6 cups cornbread, cubed (recipe on p. 9)
½ cup onion, chopped
1 cup celery, chopped
1½ tsp. sage
1¼ tsp. salt
¼ tsp. pepper
¼ cup dairy-free margarine
2 cups chicken broth (gluten free)
½ cup soy milk

BAKE cornbread. When cool, cut into cubes. Cut onion and celery, and add to cornbread. Add spices, and stir. Heat margarine on stove, and add chicken broth. When warm, add soy milk and stir. Add liquid to cornbread mixture and mix well. Pour mixture into an 8 x 8 pan, and bake at 350 degrees for 1 hour 20 minutes.

To make this recipe soy free: Substitute dairy-free margarine with an equal amount of soy-free margarine. Also substitute soy milk with an equal amount of rice or cow's milk.

E   D   S   T   N   SH   F   W   G

Chicken Salad

This is a great salad to take to a family dinner. We also make this for lunch.

4 Tbsp. sugar
2 tsp. salt
¾ cup oil
1 tsp. pepper
6 Tbsp. vinegar
2 chicken breasts, cooked and cubed
1 (16-oz.) pkg. coleslaw mix

IN a bowl, stir together sugar, salt, oil, pepper, and vinegar. Add remaining ingredients, toss, and serve.

E   D   S   T   N   SH   F   W   G

Baked Potatoes

These are great as a side to any dish and taste like a restaurant's baked potatoes.

6–8 potatoes
½ cup olive oil
¼ cup salt

WASH potatoes. Pour oil in a bowl. Rub oil over potato and sprinkle with salt. Bake in oven at 350 degrees for 1 hour.

E   D   S   T   N   SH   F   W   G

Baked Beans

This was always a favorite dish at family picnics when I was growing up. You'll soon call it a favorite too.

1½ pounds hamburger
1 onion, chopped
½ green pepper, chopped
½ cup brown sugar
1 Tbsp. mustard
½ cup ketchup
1 Tbsp. gluten- and fish-free Worcestershire sauce (optional)
½ cup water
2 large (28-oz.) cans of baked beans (gluten free)

BROWN hamburger with onion and green pepper. Add brown sugar, mustard, ketchup, Worcestershire sauce, and water. Simmer for 20 minutes and add baked beans. Then simmer for 15 minutes.

Tip: You can brown hamburger with onion and green pepper in a skillet and then put all ingredients in a slow cooker on low for 1 hour.

E   D   S   T   N   SH   F   W   G

side dishes

Mashed Potatoes

These are great as a side to any meal and, of course, for Thanksgiving dinner.

8–10 potatoes
¼ cup soy milk
1 tsp. salt

dash of pepper
3 Tbsp. dairy-free margarine

PEEL and boil potatoes for 20–25 minutes. Drain water and mash potatoes. Add soy milk, salt, pepper, and margarine. Stir.

To make this recipe soy free: Substitute dairy-free margarine with an equal amount of soy-free margarine. Also substitute soy milk with an equal amount of rice or cow's milk.

E   D   S   T   N   SH   F   W   G

Sweet Potato Bake

I brought these to a Thanksgiving meal and decided they are good any time.

1 (29-oz.) can sweet potatoes or yams
½ cup brown sugar
4 Tbsp. dairy-free margarine
marshmallows (gluten and egg free)

DRAIN sweet potatoes and pour into an 8 x 8 pan. Sprinkle brown sugar over sweet potatoes. Cut margarine into chunks and distribute over top of sweet potatoes. Bake at 350 degrees for 30 minutes. Take out of oven and sprinkle marshmallows on top. Bake until marshmallows are golden brown.

To make this recipe soy free: Substitute dairy-free margarine with an equal amount of soy-free margarine.

E   D   S   T   N   SH   F   W   G

Oven Potatoes

My kids love these potatoes! You can replace the dairy-free margarine with olive oil, if you prefer. You can also cook these in the microwave if you need them fast.

6–8 potatoes
½ cup dairy-free margarine
1½ tsp. parsley
1 tsp. salt
⅛ tsp. pepper
½ tsp. garlic salt

WASH and slice potatoes and place in an 8 x 8 pan. Put margarine over potatoes. Sprinkle all other spices over potatoes. Bake at 350 degrees for 1 hour.

To make this recipe soy free: Substitute dairy-free margarine with an equal amount of soy-free margarine or olive oil.

E   D   S   T   N   SH   F   W   G

Summer Squash

There is always plenty of squash and zucchini in the summer. We love this with any main dish.

1 small yellow squash, cut
1 small zucchini, cut
2 Tbsp. dairy-free margarine
¼ tsp. garlic powder
1 tsp. salt
⅛ tsp. pepper

WASH squash and zucchini and cut into ½-inch thick circles. Heat frying pan with margarine. Place vegetables in pan. Add garlic powder, salt, and pepper. Cook for 5 minutes on each side or until tender. Stir frequently to prevent burning.

To make this recipe soy free: Substitute dairy-free margarine with an equal amount of soy-free margarine.

E   D   S   T   N   SH   F   W   G

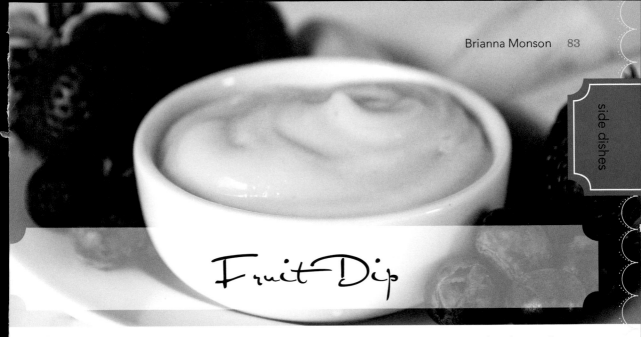

Fruit Dip

My family loves to dunk fruits in this yummy dip. They especially like to use strawberries, apples, bananas, grapes, and pineapple. If your kids won't eat fruit, they will after they try this dip!

1 (8-oz.) package dairy-free cream cheese
¾ cup sugar
1 Tbsp. orange juice, concentrate

MIX ingredients in a mixer until well blended. Pour into a bowl and serve with your favorite fruit.

E   D   S   T   N   SH   F   W   G

Green Bean Dish

This is great as a side dish for any occasion.

½ onion, chopped
2 Tbsp. dairy-free margarine
12 slices bacon (dairy and gluten free), cooked and crumbled
5 (14.5-oz.) cans green beans (French style)
1½ tsp. garlic powder
salt and pepper, to taste

SAUTÉ onion in margarine. Cook bacon. Place green beans in a slow cooker. Add onion and bacon on top of green beans. Sprinkle garlic powder, salt, and pepper over the top, and cook on low for 1 hour.

To make this recipe soy free: Substitute dairy-free margarine with an equal amount of soy-free margarine.

E   D   S   T   N   SH   F   W   G

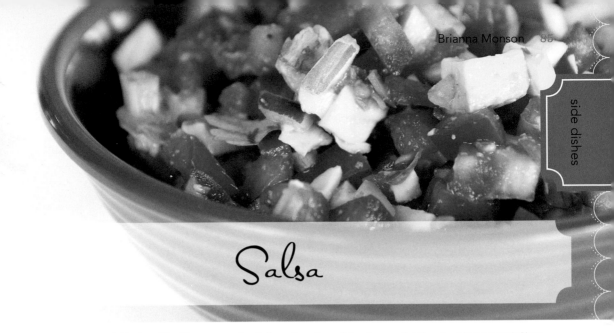

Salsa

This salsa is very addicting. You'll never go back to a store-bought salsa again! Try doubling or tripling the recipe.

3 small tomatoes, diced
1 cup red onion, diced
3 green onions, cut fine
3 Tbsp. cilantro, cut up
½ avocado, cut up
½ lime, cut in half and squeezed
1 tsp. salt
¼ tsp. pepper
¼ tsp. garlic powder

WASH all produce. Cut up vegetables and place in a medium-sized bowl. Add salt, pepper and garlic powder. Stir, and serve with corn chips or corn tortillas.

E   D   S   T   N   SH   F   W   G

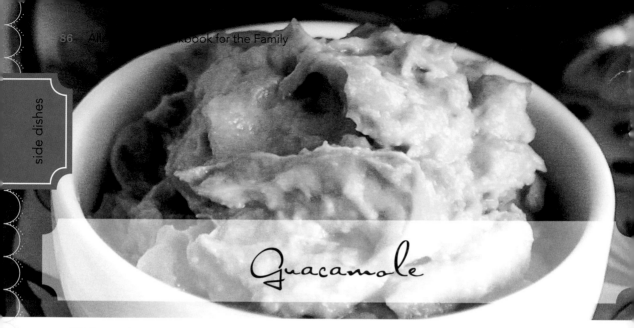

Guacamole

We love to have this with our tacos and also as a snack with chips and salsa.

2 avocados
2 Tbsp. onion, diced
2 Tbsp. tomato, diced
¼ tsp. salt
½ Tbsp. lime juice

PEEL and pit avocados. Place in a bowl and mash well. Add diced onions and tomatoes, and mix. Add salt and lime juice. Stir and enjoy.

E   D   S   T   N   SH   F   W   G

Snacks

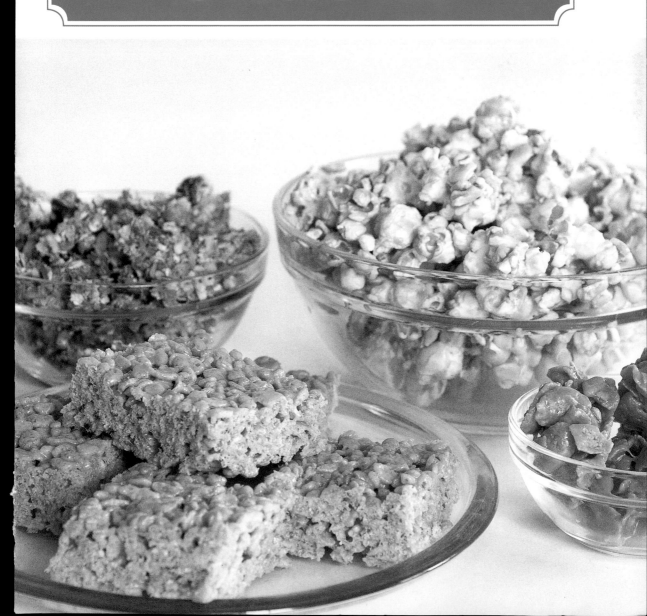

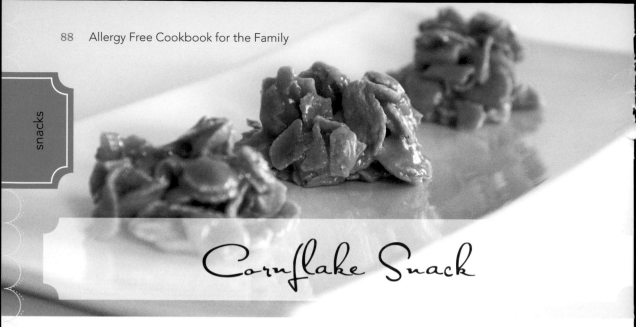

Cornflake Snack

These are great snacks for after school because they are quick to make and kids love to eat them.

½ cup soy nut butter
½ cup sugar
½ cup corn syrup
3 cups cornflakes (gluten free)

COMBINE soy nut butter, sugar, and corn syrup in a saucepan on medium. Stir until it begins to boil. Remove from heat and stir in cornflakes. Spoon mixture onto wax paper, and let sit 5 minutes to cool.

E   D   S   T   N   SH   F   W   G

Granola

My family eats this up so fast. It's great as a snack or for a breakfast cereal.

2½ cups quick oats
½ tsp. salt
1½ cups coconut flakes (optional)*
1 tsp. vanilla (gluten free)
1/3 cup maple syrup (dairy and gluten free)
1 cup rice cereal (gluten free)
¾ cup raisins

COMBINE oats, salt, coconut flakes, vanilla, syrup, and rice cereal in a bowl and mix. Pour mixture onto a greased cookie sheet and bake at 350 degrees for 20–30 minutes. Cool and stir in raisins. Store in an airtight container.

To make this recipe gluten free: Substitute quick oats with an equal amount of gluten-free oats.

*If you suffer from a tree nut allergy, you may need to avoid coconut. If so, just leave the coconut out of the recipe.

E   D   S   T   N   SH   F   W   G

Granola Bars

I created these granola bars so my kids could have a fun yet healthy treat. They turned out great, and my kids continually ask me to make them.

½ cup dairy-free margarine
1 cup brown sugar
¼ cup sugar
2 Tbsp. honey
2 cups quick oats
1 cup coconut flakes (optional)*
½ tsp. baking soda
¼ tsp. salt
½ cup dairy-free chocolate chips (optional)

IN a saucepan, heat margarine and sugars until boiling, stirring continuously. Remove from heat, add remaining ingredients, and stir. Pour onto a greased cookie sheet. This will spread when cooked. Cook at 325 degrees for 20 minutes. Remove from the oven and let cool for 10 minutes. Cut into squares, and store in an airtight container.

To make this recipe soy free: Substitute dairy-free margarine with an equal amount of soy free margarine.
To make this recipe gluten free: Substitute quick oats with an equal amount of gluten-free oats.

*If you suffer from a tree nut allergy, you may need to avoid coconut. If so, just leave the coconut out of the recipe.

E   D   S   T   N   SH   F   W   G

Sweet Snack

Here is a variation to the traditional treat. My kids and I came up with it together and really like it.

2 Tbsp. dairy-free margarine
2 cups colored marshmallows (gluten and egg free)
2 cups corn or rice cereal (gluten free)
¼ cup raisins

HEAT margarine and marshmallows in a pan until melted. Take off stove, and add cereal and raisins. Mix together. Store in an airtight container.

To make this recipe soy free: Substitute dairy-free margarine with an equal amount of soy-free margarine.

E   D   S   T   N   SH   F   W   G

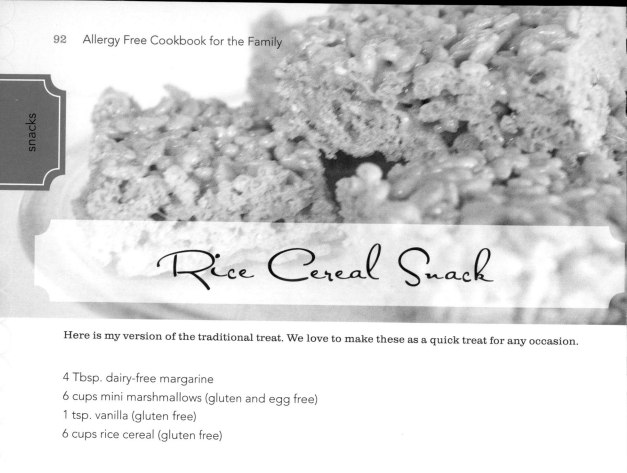

Rice Cereal Snack

Here is my version of the traditional treat. We love to make these as a quick treat for any occasion.

4 Tbsp. dairy-free margarine
6 cups mini marshmallows (gluten and egg free)
1 tsp. vanilla (gluten free)
6 cups rice cereal (gluten free)

MELT margarine and marshmallows on stove. Add vanilla and stir. Remove from heat, and stir in rice cereal. Spoon mixture out into a greased 9 x 13 pan. Let cool and cut into squares. Store in an airtight container.

Tip: You can add a few drops of food coloring to make these pretty for a holiday treat.
To make this recipe soy free: Substitute dairy-free margarine with an equal amount of soy-free margarine.

E   D   S   T   N   SH   F   W   G

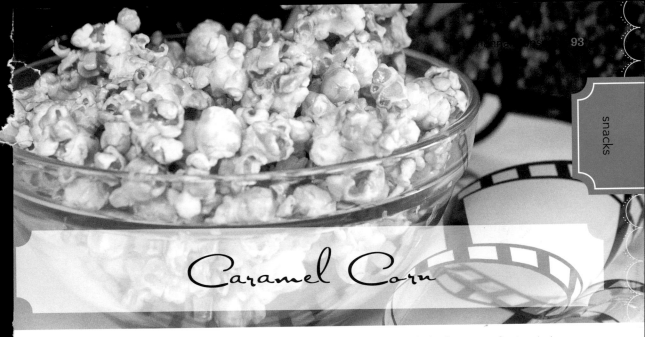

Caramel Corn

Everyone loves it when I make this for our family movie night treat. This is also a popular treat at our family reunions. You can easily make big batches for any big group.

½ cup dairy-free margarine
1 cup brown sugar
½ cup corn syrup
16 cups popped popcorn

MELT margarine in saucepan. Add brown sugar and corn syrup, and bring to a boil. Pour over popcorn, and stir well.

To make this recipe soy free: Substitute dairy-free margarine with an equal amount of soy-free margarine.

E   D   S   T   N   SH   F   W   G

Popcorn Snack

The kids love helping with this treat because they get to choose the color of the gelatin. It's fun to make a batch for a treat with friends or for a party.

½ cup dairy-free margarine
½ cup corn syrup
⅔ cup sugar
1 (3-oz.) package flavored gelatin
12 cups popped popcorn

ON stove melt margarine. (While heating margarine, you can make popcorn.) Add corn syrup, sugar, and gelatin to margarine, and bring to a slow boil. Spread popcorn onto a cookie sheet. Pour sugar mixture over popcorn. Let cool and enjoy!

Tip: To make popcorn balls, wet hands and form popcorn mixture into balls. Set aside. Wrap with plastic wrap.

To make this recipe soy free: Substitute dairy-free margarine with an equal amount of soy-free margarine.

E   D   S   T   .N   SH   F   W   G

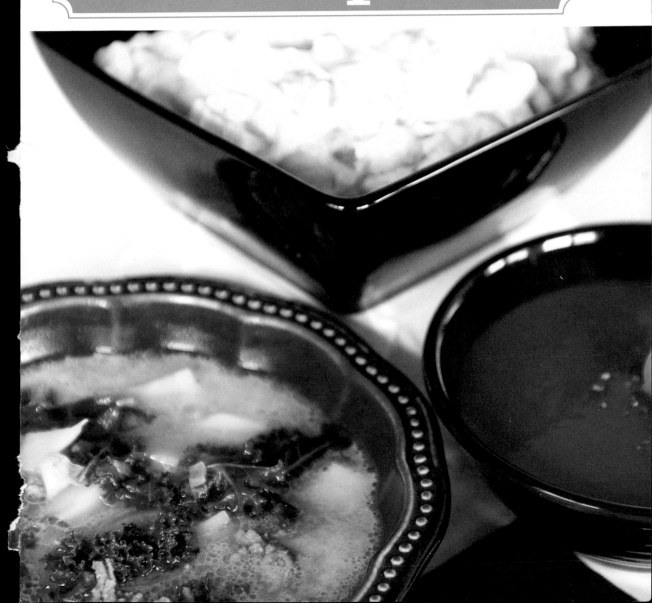

Soups

Ham and Bean Soup

When we have ham for dinner, I like to make this with the leftover ham. Don't forget to make the cornbread muffins from p. 9 to go along with it.

1 ham bone
1 lb. ham, cut up
6–8 cups water
1 (16-oz.) package white northern beans
6 slices bacon (dairy and gluten free), cooked and diced
½ onion, chopped
2 tsp. salt
1 tsp. pepper

COMBINE all ingredients in a pot and cook for 2–2½ hours until beans are soft.

E   D   S   T   N   SH   F   W   G

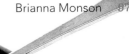

soups

Tomato Soup

I had to create a tomato soup recipe because I grew up on tomato soup and loved it. It's also good to make for casseroles that call for tomato soup.

1 (6-oz.) can tomato paste
1¼ cups water
3 Tbsp. sugar
½ tsp. salt
¼ cup soy milk

COMBINE all ingredients in a saucepan and heat through.

To make this recipe soy free: Substitute soy milk with an equal amount of rice or cow's milk.

E   D   S   T   N   SH   F   W   G

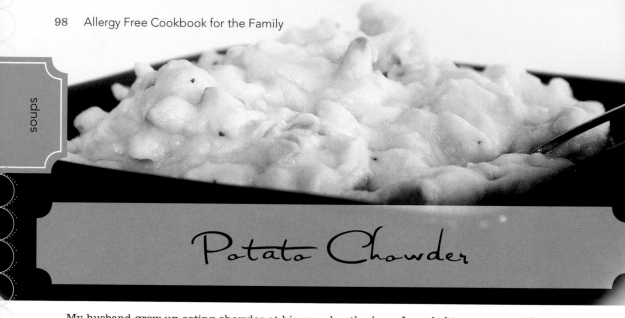

Potato Chowder

My husband grew up eating chowder at his grandmother's, so I needed to come up with a chowder that my son could eat too.

1½ cups onion, chopped
¼ cup dairy-free margarine
½ cup celery, chopped
½ cup carrots, chopped
2½ cups potatoes, cubed
3 Tbsp. water

1 Tbsp. salt
½ tsp. pepper
½ cup rice flour
4 cups soy milk
1 cup water

SAUTÉ onion in pot with margarine. Add celery, carrots, and potatoes to onions, and cook for 10 minutes. Add remaining ingredients and bring to a slow boil, stirring frequently. Cover, and cook for 1 hour, stirring occasionally.

Tip: If you can have clams, add a can of clams for clam chowder.
To make this recipe soy free: Substitute dairy-free margarine with an equal amount of soy-free margarine. Also substitute soy milk with an equal amount of rice or cow's milk.

E   D   S   T   N   SH   F   W   G

Chicken or Turkey Soup

My son says he loves the soup that I cook in the big pot. He loves the smell of it cooking and thinks it's so much better than the store-bought kind.

4 cups water

2 (32-oz.) boxes chicken broth (gluten free)

4 cups chicken or turkey, cooked and cut up

2 cups celery, cut up

3 cups carrots, sliced

1 cup onion, chopped

½ Tbsp. salt

2 tsp. garlic salt

1 Tbsp. basil

½ tsp. pepper

1⅓ cups instant rice

POUR water and chicken broth into pot. Add meat and vegetables to pot. Add spices and cook for 1–1½ hours on medium. Add rice and cook 5 minutes longer.

E   D   S   T   N   SH   F   W   G

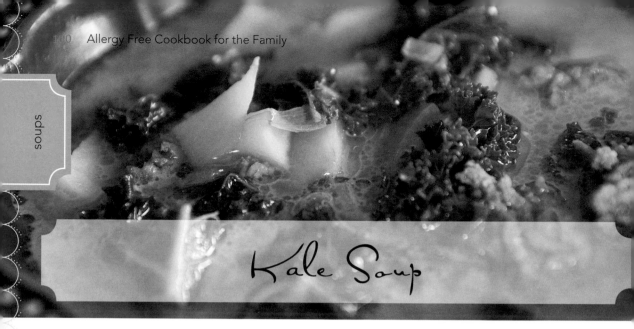

Kale Soup

I love the kale soup at my favorite restaurant, so I came up with my own version for us to enjoy at home with the whole family. I even grow kale in my garden just for this recipe.

1 onion, chopped
½ cup dairy-free margarine
6 slices bacon (dairy and gluten free), cooked and crumbled
1 cup chicken broth (gluten free)
8 cups water
4 potatoes, cubed
4 garlic cloves, minced
2 tsp. salt
¼ tsp. pepper
½ lb. hamburger
4 cups kale, chopped
1 cup dairy-free creamer

SAUTÉ onion with margarine in pot. Cook bacon and add to pot. Add broth, water, potatoes, garlic, salt, and pepper, and cook on medium-high for 20 minutes. Brown hamburger and add to pot. Wash and chop kale. Add kale and creamer to pot and cook another 5 minutes on low.

E   D   S   T   N   SH   F   W   G

Hamburger Stew

This is a great stew for a cold or rainy day. It's easy to make and smells great while it simmers on the stove.

1 lb. hamburger

1 cup onion, chopped

1 cup celery, chopped

1 cup carrots, cut up

1 (14.5-oz.) can diced tomatoes

1 Tbsp. dried parsley

1 tsp. basil

1 bay leaf

1 (32-oz.) box chicken or beef broth (gluten free)

2 cups water

BROWN hamburger. While hamburger is cooking, cut up vegetables and place in a pot on stove. Add hamburger and remaining ingredients and simmer for 1 hour.

E   D   S   T   N   SH   F   W   G

Resources

BE sure to do your research so you know if an ingredient will be safe for you. Everyone has different dietary/allergy needs, so please double-check before you use an ingredient. Here's a list of places to find ingredients or specialty foods.

www.allergiesandme.com
www.authenticfoods.com
www.bobsredmill.com
www.earthbalancenatural.com
www.ener-g.com
www.enjoylifefoods.com
www.freefrommarket.com
www.glutenfreemall.com
www.glutenfreeoats.com
www.pacificfoods.com
www.san-j.com
www.silksoymilk.com
www.smartbalance.com
www.spectrumorganics.com
www.tofutti.com
www.wholefoodsmarket.com

HERE is a list of places to find helpful information on food allergies and celiac disease.

www.aaaai.org
www.allergicchild.com
www.allergymoms.com
www.anaphylaxis.org
www.foodallergy.org
www.foodallergybuzz.com
www.faiusa.org
www.foodfacts.com
www.kidswithfoodallergies.org

Recipe Index

About the Author

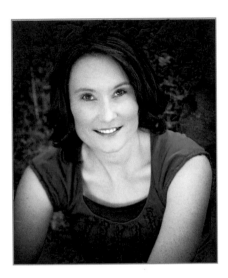

BRIANNA Monson was born in Oregon and grew up in Washington. She played collegiate golf for two years and still enjoys playing when she gets the chance. She graduated with a bachelor's in elementary education. She currently lives in Washington State with her husband and two children. Her children were born with severe food allergies, and due to this challenge, she spends a lot of time in the kitchen preparing special foods. This soon became a passion, and she began experimenting to prepare foods they could tolerate and the whole family would enjoy. This has been a pleasant experience as she sees the smiles on her children's faces while they help in the kitchen. Brianna truly believes that those with food allergies should and can be included in family and social gatherings involving food.